Also authored by
Daniel Weber, PhD MSc

Inflammation and the Seven Stochastic Events of Cancer

Introduction to Integrative Oncology: Herbs, Compounds and Supplements in the Treatment of Cancer

Dui Yao: the Art of Formula Construction

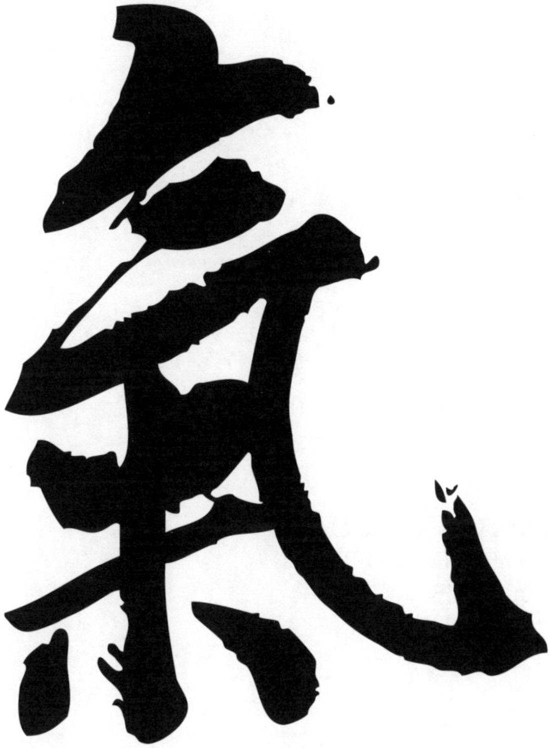

MODERN & ANCIENT

**"No Movements of qi are Identical;
Ancient and Modern Times Differ;
Ancient Formulas are Helpless for Modern Diseases."**

Zhang Yuan-su 1151- 1234 C.E.
(THE JIN-YUAN MEDICAL REFORMS)

Published and distributed by:
PANAXEA PUBLISHING
A division of CHM/RD Pty Ltd
74-78 Brandling St
Alexandria NSW 2015
Sydney, Australia

www.panaxea.com

US Distribution by Redwing Book Company
First Edition, May 2010
ISBN: 978-0-646-50961-7

Cover and Page Design: Fabien Rebuffel • www.cidfabylon.com

Printed in China

DISCLAIMER
Traditional complementary and integrative medicine (TCIM) is a professional medicine. Laypersons interested in availing themselves of the treatments described in this book should seek out a qualified professional practitioner.

FOREWORD

Western scientific medicine is based upon a culture, which experienced the 'Age of Enlightenment' and the 'Age of Reason' as well as the rational schools of Greek philosophy. Traditional Chinese medicine is based upon the cultural values that arise within their cultural experiences, emphasising family and leadership filial loyalties. Western understandings of Chinese culture and medicine are often viewed through the lens of Western values. Culture refers to integrated patterns of human behaviour that include the language, thoughts, communications, actions, customs, beliefs, values, and institutions of racial, ethnic, religious, or social groups. The professional culture of medicine can be viewed as the language, thought processes, styles of communication, customs, and beliefs that often characterise the profession of medicine (Kleinman, 1978). Also, the way in which physicians conceptualise health is another example of the physician's culture. This is referred to as the explanatory model and when used in reference to patients, explanatory models describe how patients interpret the meaning of an illness and the impact that it has on their ability to function (Kleinman, 1987). A culture's idiom of distress not only influences clinical care and but also has a great impact on medical theory and the formalised "voice of medicine". For example, modern Chinese and Japanese medical theoreticians speak of the liver and the heart more sensitive to emotional issues than other organs (Kaptchuk, 1987).

Qi, Shen, San Jiao and Blood amongst others, are not things but multi-level integrated systems, which are not fixed, ever adapting and changing. Organs [Liver, Kidney, Spleen etc] are not things but systems involving physical organs [sometimes], meridians [spheres of influence], the CNS, ANS, endocrine and immune systems and their interactive relationships.

These are vertical systems. Yuan qi or primordial-qi, also called primary qi is the most essential qi in the body and the vital foundation of life. Primordial qi is mainly generated from the kidney-qi of the parents during pregnancy. The power and quantity of primordial qi is therefore fixed at birth. Primordial qi contributes to the general functions of qi, such as propelling, warming, protecting, fixating & transforming.

Ancient traditional Chinese medicine (TCM) has effectively relied on the theory of yin/yang balance in diagnoses and treatments of diseases and disorders for more than 2000 years. However, in eastern society, yin-yang is regarded as an incomprehensible ideology without definite physical meaning but it may have a physiological basis. The yin-yang balance is anti-oxidation/oxidation balance with yin representing anti-oxidation and yang as oxidation. The proposal is partially supported by the fact that the yin-tonic traditional Chinese herbs have, on average, about six times more antioxidant activity and polyphenolic contents than the yang-tonic herbs (Ou et al, 2003). The 'Yin-Yang' theory is an ancient Chinese philosophy that underlies the practice of traditional Chinese medicine. Although yang-tonic herbs tend to boost body function possibly through enhancing the mitochondrial oxidative processes, the yin property (i.e. antioxidant potential) of these herbs can also play a role in safeguarding mitochondrial adenosine triphosphate (ATP) generation. The pharmacological basis of 'yang-invigoration' by Chinese tonic herbs might be due primarily to the enhancement of mitochondrial ATP generation (Ko et al, 2004). Chinese herbs, classified into 4 properties (hot, warm, cold and cool) of TCM, were analysed for their ability to exhibit antioxidant action, to enhance glucose uptake by murine microglia N9 cells, and to influence neurotransmitter norepinephrine (NE) release from PC12 cells. A generally protective effect of both hot/warm-natured and cold/cool-natured herbs against H2O2-induced N9 cell death, partially by elevating superoxide dismutase (SOD) activity.

Glucose uptake was elevated after treatment with some hot/warm-natured herbs. In addition, most herbs with hot/warm nature tended to stimulate NE release, while such stimulatory effect was not observed in the herbs with cold/cool nature. Two cold/cool-natured herbs, huang lian (Rhizoma coptidis) and huang qin (Radix scutellariae), even significantly suppressed the release. These results suggest that the distinct abilities of Chinese herbs to regulate neural cell functions appear to be correlated with their natures identified in traditional TCM theory, and may be a useful guide for their utility in neural degenerative diseases. Hot-natured herbs enhanced cellular antioxidant status and stimulated neural transmitter norepinephrine release. Glucose uptake was upregulated in response to several typical hot-natured herbs. Cold-natured herbs, which possessed greater antioxidant properties, tended to suppress norepinephrine production, thereby attenuating over-reactive neural cells (Liu Y-Q et al, 2008).

Psychophysiology and psychoneuroimmunology are Western disciplines attempting to formalise the Chinese and other traditional medical / spiritual understandings. Psyche is the process of transformation, of growth and change and emotion is not a thing but a neurophysiological response to stimuli, while a feeling is the conscious recognition of an emotional event. The body is much more than the sum of its parts. Our being does not stop at the skin. We are the sum of all experiences and people. Modern approaches to traditional medicine is best served by a systems biology (SB) method and SB is a general trend of contemporary scientific development, which describe the interconnectivity and interdependence of the components of the system and which recognise that new properties of systems are revealed as increasing levels of complexity are studied. SB is 'studying biology as an integrated system of genetic, protein, metabolite, cellular and pathway events that are in flux and interdependent'. This does not imply that all elements need to be measured for systems studies but that systems thinking and systems-based analytical strategies are key (van der Greef et al 2004). TCM can be considered as an ancient and classical paradigm of systems biology. In TCM, diagnosis and medication are based on "Syndrome" (ZHENG), which can be regarded as a profile of symptom combination, or clinical phenotypes, such as Cold or Hot Syndrome, and "Hot medication curing Cold Syndrome" is a standard therapeutic guide line (Ma et al, 2010).

Anxiety is the psychophysiologic signal that the stress response has been initiated. The stress response can be viewed as an interactional process that causes psychophysiologic reactions that are immediate and can occur up to and including physiologic events 3 weeks after confrontation with the stressor. The literature suggests that neuroendocrine alterations in response to confrontation with a stressor may influence immunocompetence. Coping strategies that fall into four categories: behavioural, physical, cognitive, and emotional (Robinson, 1990).

From: Cozolino 2006

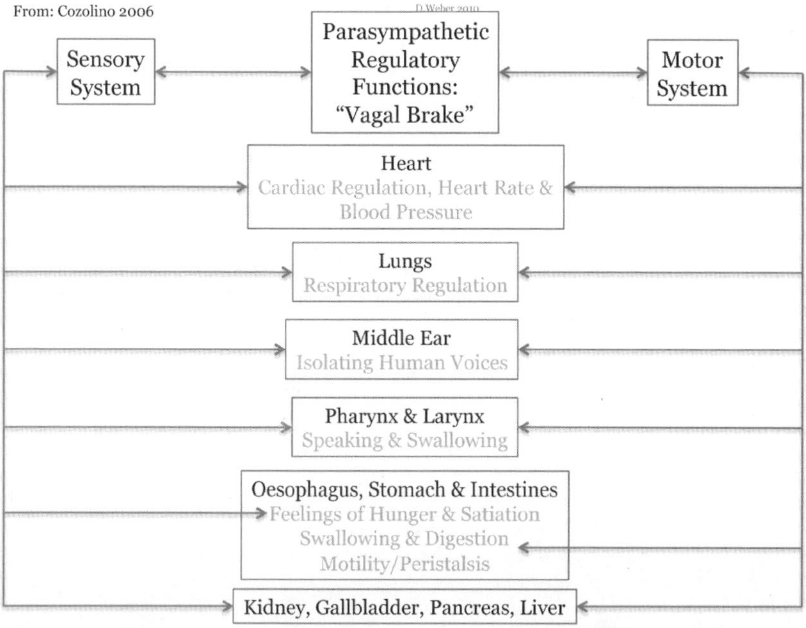

The Vagal system has afferent and efferent branches to control organ function as well as receive information from the organs. This ensures physical and psychological communication to activate brain/body responses to stimuli.

CHAPTER CONTENTS

INTRODUCTION

Mood disorders, which include depression, anxiety as well as general psychological malaise and stress is an increasingly common problem in the clinic. Orthodox medical approaches focus upon talk treatments; counselling, psychotherapy and behavioural modification or psychotropic drugs to restore neurotransmitter function. This approach seems to be a result of the very deep Cartesian split our culture makes around the body and mind. Traditional medicines see psychological problems as just an aspect of imbalance in the whole being, the body and mind just parts of a continuum. Treatments focus upon restoring the balance within the whole being, which includes the physical manifestation, the emotional/perceptive system and the cultural idiom of the time.

Traditional Chinese Medicine (TCM) uses a system of *Pattern Recognition* to identify the nature of the imbalance regardless of the name or symptom. This subtle but highly efficacious diagnostic system is friendlier to clinical medicine but more complex in application. Recently Western understandings of the function of the central nervous system (CNS), autonomic nervous system (ANS) and the endocrine system and their interaction begins to show a deeper appreciation of the unity of the whole being and a breakdown of the Cartesian bias. Of particular interest is the vagal nerve and Porges' theory of the Social Nervous System. The contrast between certain features in TCM with Western understandings of the ANS are of interest, particularly the TCM Triple Warmer theory with Polyvagal Tone theory.

Emotions and Their Experience

How does one make a distinction between feelings and emotions? John Wellwood, a contemporary Buddhist psychotherapist approaches the problem of emotion from a complementary position (Wellwood, 1992).

In Western culture we have a history of treating emotions with suspicion and fear, as something that overcomes us and is separate from our rational self. The "passions" have usually been viewed as our "lower nature", from Plato onward. Viewing the source of the passions as Freud did, as an Id, a primitive chaos, it makes it more difficult to understand emotions and accept them as part of us. This view of emotions as primitive and alien seems to be a classic Western way of separating ourselves from them. This is in sharp contrast to the Chinese approach, which views emotions as a somatic event, a lived experience.

The spectrum of feelings range from the purely physical to the largely mental and this spectrum can be seen as what Wellwood called:

- the spectrum of felt energy
- emotions
- feelings
- felt senses
- basic aliveness (qi)

All our feelings and emotions grow out of a basic life stream coursing through us called qi, this basic aliveness is a wholesome feeling persisting beneath all the ups and downs of circumstances.

Our basic aliveness is also the source of our sensitivity and tenderness. Because we are fundamentally open and receptive to life, we are vulnerable. Our soft skin, the intricate workings of our senses, brain, and nervous system are all geared toward letting the world in. Feeling and emotion are what arise in response to letting the world in.

Between the pure aliveness and the specific feelings and emotions we are most familiar with, we have more global kinds of "felt senses" about the life situations we are in. Because a felt sense includes many different aspects of how we relate to a situation, it may seem vague or fuzzy at first, appearing for instance, as a tightness in the chest or a heaviness in the stomach. This is often called 'mood'.

In contrast to a felt sense, feelings, such as sadness, gladness, or anger are relatively familiar and more recognisable. Feelings give us context for the current human/social environment. Feelings are internal clues as to a social situation, giving information on the group's psychological construction. In Japan and China one is expected to know the operative soma/emotio state of the group. In the Orient the somatic experience of feelings is as universal as it is hidden and expression of emotion is seen as a loss of social harmony.

Emotions are a more intense form of feelings as they direct behaviour and build upon responses from others. They are biologically driven, cross-cultural responses to environmental stimuli. The feeling of sadness may build into grief; the feeling of irritation can become a fierce rage. The distinguishing characteristic of emotion is that it dominates our attention and cannot be ignored, while feeling can remain in the background of awareness. Emotions carry value; they are 'good' or 'bad'. Emotions are also cultural, what we call anger differs between various cultures and are a learned phenomena whereas 'felt sense' is organic and evolutionary.

Candace Pert (1988) describes the theory of how the "body-mind" functions as a single psychosomatic network of information molecules; thoughts, feelings, sensations and the biological feedback of digestion, heart function and elimination are just one. The spectrum from aliveness to emotion is one of increasing cognition.

Emotions and Self

The Buddhist definition of ego as "holding on to ourselves" and controlling our experience helps us understand why it is so hard to let ourselves feel our emotions and let them be. We usually try to keep them from flowing through us because they threaten the control we try to maintain. When we recognise that somatic awareness is a process of experiencing the pre personal non-self (MU) we can understand the Chinese system of yin/yang. The biological self is posited in a continuum with the psychological self. This yin/yang continuum does not however contain egoic self which is purely reification i.e. habit of Mind.

All of this can be summed up as "MU". This also speaks much more comprehensively and creatively to the theories postulated by Melanie Klein and the *Object Relations School of Psychoanalysis.* The object self is a construct or I create I to have a continual and ongoing Self. We desperately fear losing our 'Self'.

Feelings; East and West

The very experience of selfhood itself is different in China and in the West. The embodiment and manifestation are particular to each culture and to each time. Emotions and affect are ways in which sensitivity to our states of being and behaviour differs between East and West. This necessarily has a tremendous impact on how illness and health manifest. The Chinese concept of person contrasts sharply with the Western concept of personality; The concept of personality puts emphasis on what goes on in the individual's psyche including his /her unconscious (Kaptchuk, 1988).

The contemporary Western patient tends to experience selfhood as "individual-centred" and monitors his changing states in intensely personal and existential terms, while the contemporary Chinese patient tends to view selfhood as "situation-centred" and illness and health in physical terms. The traditional Chinese 'self' appears to be relatively more orientated toward the significant others, rather than toward the individual self.

Our Western sense of self was developed in the brief period from the 5th to the 3rd century B.C.E. in Greece. Homer's description of the hero differs considerably from expressions made by Aristophanes or Sophocles a few centuries later. Aristotle developed a physiology of the mind based on four humours - *Blood, Mucus,* and *Yellow* and *Black Bile.* Different balances of these humours gave rise to different states of mind. Aristotle also saw the soul as an organic life force, which in 'dilutes' form gave the simple awareness of lower animals, and in concentrated or elevated form, gave the self-conscious and the rational awareness of humans.

Aristotle's theories about the vital fluids became part of the Western thought through the medical writings of Galen, the second century Greek physician. While Plato's model became entwined with Christian belief to become the West's dominant theory of the mind, Aristotle's idea of a surging life-force and four bodily humours gave physical explanation of the mind that complemented Plato's metaphysical idea of mankind poised half-way between the animal and the divine. Plato's separations and distinctions placed the body in the animal realm and the mind in the higher, purer realms.

RATIONAL MIND	(HIGHER SELF)
HIGHER EMOTION	(HUMAN SELF)
LOWER EMOTION	(ANIMAL NATURE)

This model was adapted and used by Freud:

SUPER EGO
EGO
ID

Medical Philosophy

Chinese medical philosophy began to create a model of 'man' that was dynamic and interactive with both the social and physical environment. The philosophical aspects of Chinese medicine depend upon all three streams of religious thought. In Confucianism, the order and importance of secular life gave rise to professional conduct and standards, which lifted medicine from its shamanistic roots. In Taoism, the mystery and the appreciation of yin/yang prevented a narcissistic indulgence in human centeredness and was essentially ecological. In Buddhism, the nature of emptiness (MU) began a deep phenomenalistic philosophy allowing synthetic thinking. These three religious philosophies gave the discipline a solid empirical basis for developing a viable holistic medicine.

The clinical approach in Oriental medicine recognises the continuum and interaction of the psyche and soma. The methodology has always taken into account the psychosomatic truth that psychological and physiological processes are interactive and have shared clinical significance. For example, on a very simple level, Oriental medicine can see anxiety and heart palpitations, fear and sweating, revulsion and nausea, anger and changes in metabolism, and despair and sighing as being emotional and physical concomitants of a singe yin-yang manifestation. Nevertheless, contemporary Eastern and Western people tend to experience different ends of this continuum in their lives.

Medicine as Culture

Culture refers to integrated patterns of human behaviour that include the language, thoughts, communications, actions, customs, beliefs, values, and institutions of racial, ethnic, religious, or social groups. The professional culture of medicine can be viewed as the language, thought processes, styles of communication, customs, and beliefs that often characterise the profession of medicine. Also, the way in which physicians conceptualise health is another example of the physician's culture. This is referred to as the explanatory model and when used in reference to patients, explanatory models describe how patients interpret the meaning of an illness and the impact that it has on their ability to function (Kleinman, 1978; Kleinman, 1987).

Western scientific medicine or rational medicine is based upon a culture, which experienced the 'Age of Enlightenment' and the 'Age of Reason' as well as the rational schools of Greek philosophy. Traditional Chinese medicine or empirical medicine is based upon the cultural values that arise within their experiences, emphasising family and leadership filial loyalties, social ecology and interdependence.

Rational and empirical medicines differ in how they developed their ideas. In rational medicine, the emphasis is on deductive logic and in empirical medicine the emphasis is on practical experience. However, the difference is only in emphasis, as both schools use logic and experience, only in different degrees (Coulter, 1994a). Rational medicine attempts to be deductive and while empirical medicine has always been in the minority when compared to the dominant school of rational medicine, the relative influence of both has varied through history (ibid).

Empirical physicals must take into account the experiences about the circumstances and the individuality of the patient [the idiosyncrasies] without sacrificing the particular to the general and granting primary status to phenomena (Reale, 1990). Perhaps the reason empiricism has always been in the minority is because it is harder to do. Empiricism is vitalistic, individualises the treatment to the patient and is oriented towards treating the patient's underlying condition. Rational medicine, in contrast, is mechanistic, disease rather than patient oriented (Coulter, 1994b).

Rational and empirical medicines are not opposites but reside on a spectrum, with rational medicine delving deeper into the molecular/chemical nature of disease, while empirical medicine recognises individual variations, the epigenetic variation of a disease and is patient oriented.

Autonomic Nervous System

The autonomic nervous system (ANS) (or visceral nervous system) is the part of the peripheral nervous system that acts as a control system, maintaining homeostasis in the body. These activities are generally performed without conscious control. The ANS affects heart rate, digestion, respiration rate, salivation, perspiration, and diameter of the pupils, micturition, and sexual arousal. Whereas most of its actions are involuntary, some, such as breathing, work in tandem with the conscious mind.

The ANS is divided into 2 functions:

1. The Sympathetic Nervous System (SNS), which initiates the stress response, the fight/flight syndrome.
2. The Parasympathetic Nervous System (PNS), which induces the relaxation response.

To these traditional two ANS functions we can add others, the vagus and enteric systems. Porges (1995) has shown clear evidence that the third, more modern branch of the ANS; the vagus nerve is a survival value specific to more sophisticated animals especially primates. "Social Nervous System" is the proposed term for this third branch of the ANS.

Dysregulation of this critical balance between the differing functions of the ANS is clearly responsible for a number of psycho-physical disorders. The hyper functioning of the SNS, will in general terms create restlessness, aggression, palpitations and suspicion. Hyper activity of the PNS will cause withdrawal, lack of interest and anhedonia. In a recent study on sleep and mood it was found that both depression and worry (anxiety) before sleep shift balance of ANS towards sympathetic dominance during sleep (Yoshino and Matsuoka, 2008).

Depression has been shown to directly affect the ANS and increase the risk of coronary heart disease (CHD). Depression is a risk factor for medical morbidity and mortality in patients with CHD and dysregulation of the autonomic nervous system (ANS) may explain why depressed patients are at increased risk (Carney, Freedland and Veith, 2005). Some of the earliest evidence of ANS dysregulation in depression was found in studies of medically well patients with major depressive disorder. These studies found elevated levels of plasma and urinary catecholamines, primarily norepinephrine (NE), in depressed patients compared with controls (Esler et al, 1982).

The relationship between psychological distress and angina on electrocardiogram (ECG) abnormalities was examined in a cross-sectional community study of 15,406 men and women. The associations were particularly strong for angina with and without ECG abnormalities. Psychological distress was associated with CHD morbidity in men, in fully adjusted analysis but not women. Psychological distress is associated with an increased 5-year risk of CHD mortality and morbidity in men (Rasul et al, 2003).

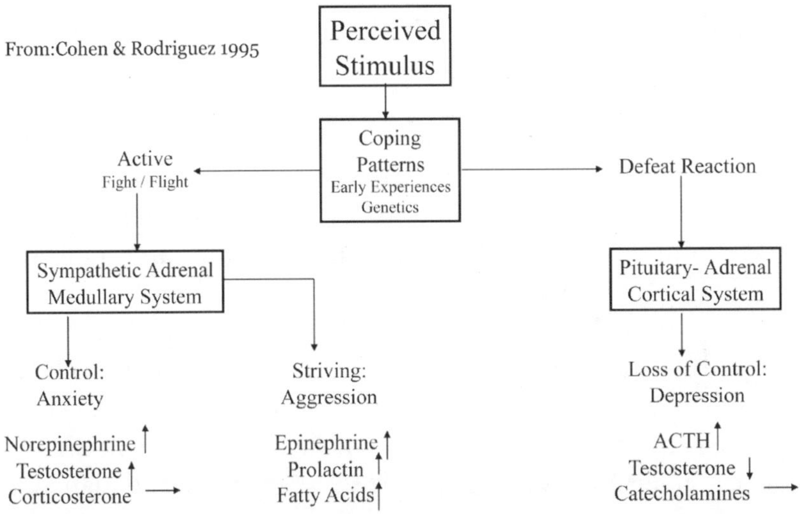

Sympathetic Adrenal-Medullary (SAM) System

The three coping patterns are dependant upon genetic predisposition, early childhood experiences and the level and persistence of the threat. The SAM system activates the neuro-endocrine system to manage perceived danger.

Stress, Mood Disorders and ANS

When there is a perception of a real or an imagined threatening stressor, the brain initiates the stress response by triggering a series of chemical chain-reactions that prepare the body for fight or flight. This reaction is a healthy, vital defence mechanism and triggers the release of hormones that affect every organ and system of the body. The hypothalamus, a collection of tissues in the brain, which then stimulates the pituitary gland in the brain which then stimulates the adrenal gland to release cortisol and norepinephrine (NE) amongst many.

Excess cortisol in the blood interferes with mood enhancing neurotransmitter called serotonin. Disturbances in serotonin levels can be a factor in causing clinical depression and anxiety disorders as well as being linked to insomnia, obesity and increased sensitivity to pain (McCance, 1998).

The stress response hormones cause a number of other biochemical and physiological changes, which in the short term are vital, but if the stressor is chronic then these stress hormones can start to undermine wellbeing. This stress response is designed to be mainly short term. In the long term these hormones cause blood clotting to increase and blood cholesterol levels to elevate increasing the risk of many diseases such as heart disease, stroke and angina. While stress hormones stimulate the immune system immediately, they weaken it in the long term. Increases in blood pressure are another long-term effect of these stress hormones increasing the risk of stroke, heart attack and kidney disease.

Recently an interesting study reported in the Archives of General Psychiatry (Volume 63, page 824) indicates that being obese is associated with about a 25% increased risk of major depression, bipolar disorder, panic disorder, and agoraphobia.

The lifetime risk of mood disorders was 18.3% among people with a BMI below 30 and 22% among people with a BMI of 30 or above. Men and women were equally affected, despite the fact that previous research suggested the link existed only in women.

Depression clearly has a harmful effect on physical health; it also makes chronic illnesses such as diabetes, arthritis, back problems, and asthma worse (Simon et al, 2006). Clearly, from a whole being system of treatment the relationship between obesity and depression is circular; one creates the other and many of the issues revolve around gut function and the enteric hormones. A simple, yet clear sign of some mood disorder is a waist/hip ratio of more than one to one.

Stress, Depression, Anxiety and Gut Function

In healthy humans stressors have been shown to result in a characteristic stress induced slowing of gastric emptying, increase in distal colonic motility and acceleration of intestinal transit. In the most common functional gastrointestinal disorders, irritable bowel syndrome (IBS) and functional gastric disorder (FGD), persistent alterations of autonomic responsiveness is likely to play a role in altered bowel habits and alteration in gastric emptying, respectively.

Evidence for such alterations in IBS includes increased responses of distal colonic motility in response to laboratory stress and possibly food intake and delayed gastric emptying in a subset of patients.

Evidence for alterations in HPA axis function has been demonstrated in diarrhoea predominant IBS patients who showed decreased 24 hour plasma cortisol, blunted cortisol responses, and normal ACTH responses to noxious rectosigmoid distension (Mayer, 2000).

Depression has been linked with both irritable bowel syndrome and non-organic abdominal pain and while depression is common in gastrointestinal outpatients it is not always appreciated and its symptoms should be sought in all patients with bowel dysfunction and chronic abdominal pain.

The Beck Depression Inventory to screen new referrals to a general medical and gastrointestinal clinic and to a minor surgical clinic showed that 50 of 100 medical patients were rated as having some degree of depression, compared with 14 of 75 (19%) of the surgical patients in whom abdominal pain and bowel dysfunction were rare. In the medical clinic no organic disorder was detected in 64% of the depressed patients, the majority of whom presented with abdominal pain or irritable bowel syndrome (Rose et al, 1986). Orocaecal transit time (OCTT) was measured by lactulose hydrogen breath test. Whole gut transit time (WGTT) was measured by abdominal radiography.

WGTT was shorter in patients with anxiety (≈14 hours) than in patients with depression (≈49 hours). OCTT was shorter (≈60 minutes) in patients with anxiety than in patients with depression (≈110 minutes).

These objective measurements of intestinal transit in affective disorders are consistent with clinical impressions that anxiety is associated with increased bowel frequency, and depressed patients tend to be constipated; mood has an effect on intestinal motor function (Gorard et al, 1996).

The Ergotropic and Trophotropic Systems; The yin/yang of Mind/Body

The Ergotropic System (ES) mediates our so-called fight or flight responses; that is, the physiological components of our adaptation strategies to desirable or noxious stimuli in the environment. Anatomically, the ergotropic system incorporates the functions of the sympathetic nervous system (one half of the autonomic nervous system), certain of the endocrine glands, portions of the reticular activating system in the brain stem, the posterior hypothalamus, and portions of the limbic system and frontal cortex. The principle function of the ergotropic system is the control of short-range, moment-by-moment adaptation to events in the environment.

The Trophotropic System (TS) is far less dramatic in its activities, but is nonetheless the system responsible for regulating the vegetative functions, such as repair and growth of cells, digestion, relaxation, sleep, and so on. Anatomically, the trophotropic system incorporates the functions of the parasympathetic system (the other half of the autonomic nervous system), various endocrine glands, other portions of the reticular activating system, the anterior hypothalamus, and other portions of the limbic system and frontal cortex.

It is the trophotropic system that controls the somatic functions responsible for the long-term wellbeing, growth, development and longevity of the organism. This system operates to maintain the optimal internal balance of bodily functions for continued health and development of the body, and consequently of the mind (Hellhammer & Hellhammer, 2008).

The ES and TS have been described as "antagonistic" to each other. The increased activity of the one tends to produce a decreased activity in the other. This is the case because each system is physically designed to inhibit the functioning of the other under most circumstances. In excitation [anger, anxiety, fear, strong desire etc], the ergotropic system not only produces the requisite physiological, emotional and behavioural responses, it also puts a damper [via reciprocal inhibition] on the trophotropic system, which was previously sub-serving digestion and other metabolic activities. Likewise, when a person relaxes, the trophotropic system actively dampens the activity of the ergotropic system (Gellhorn, 1967).

Vagal System; Social Nervous System

Vagus nerve has its fibres distributed in the neck, thorax and abdomen. Generally speaking, vagus nerve has motor fibres to the bronchial tree, inhibitory fibres to the heart, motor fibres to the oesophagus, stomach, small intestine and gall passages, and secretory fibres to the stomach and pancreas.

Activation or deactivation of vagus nerve will typically lead to the changes in heart rate, blood pressure, gastrointestinal smooth muscle movement and secretions of digestive glands.

Vagal reflex control circuits in the dorsal vagal complex of the brainstem provide overall coordination over digestive functions of the stomach, small intestine and pancreas (Rogers et al, 1996) and the vagus nerve plays a counter-inflammatory role in acute colitis and IBD (Ghia et al, 2006)

Stimulation of the vagus nerve increased heart rate (Ng et al, 2001) and the vagus nerve exerts a profound influence on the heart, regulating the heart rate and rhythm. An extensive vagal innervation of the cardiac ventricles and the central origin are numerous, and their distribution within the nucleus ambiguus and dorsal motor nucleus of the vagus is similar to that of neurons innervating other cardiac targets, such as the sino-atrial node (Standish et al, 1994).

It has now been over a decade since Porges (1995) first advanced Polyvagal Theory. In that time, the theory has lent coherence to a wide range of clinical observations among a diverse array of psychiatric conditions spanning both the internalising and externalising spectra. The theory has provided unique insights into the role of emotional dysregulation in psychopathology, and into the development of aberrant patterns of autonomic nervous system functioning in numerous clinical syndromes that before were considered unrelated (Beauchaine, 2008).

Stress

Stress is a normal response to a demand for adaptation and stress is an integral part of life. It allows the body to adjust or adapt to a multitude of positive or negative events that are experienced. Stress shows up as various physical, cognitive, and emotional reactions. The ability to adapt to new situations depends on the individual's personality, beliefs, past and current experiences and support network (MSSS 200). Stimuli that are interpreted by the brain as extreme or threatening, regardless of their modality, elicit an immediate stereotypic response characterised by enhanced cognition, affective immobility, vigilance, autonomic arousal and a global catabolic state. The brain differentially activates a subset of vagal and sacral parasympathetic efferents that mediate the gut responses to stress (Habib et al, 2001). The vagal nerve also activates heart rate, respiration, epigastric motility and expression. Vagal tone is proposed as a novel index of stress vulnerability and reactivity with applications in all branches of medicine and measurement of cardiac vagal tone is a method to assess on an individual basis both the stress response and the vulnerability to stress (Porges, 1992). Cardiac vagal tone is proposed as a novel index of stress and stress vulnerability in mammals (Porges, 1995).

Vagal Tone is a critical component in how stress is managed. Higher vagal tone is a sign of psycho-physical competence.

Higher Vagal Tone:
Self Regulation
Self Soothing
Control of Emotions (not suppression)
Reliable Autonomic Response
Suppression of Heart Rate

Enhanced Attention
Positive Social response
Increased Behavioural Engagement
Consistent Caretaking/ Secure Attachment

Lower Vagal Tone:
Irritability
Behavioural Problems
Emotional Dysregulation
Distractibility
Hyper-reactivity to Environmental & Visceral Stimuli
Withdrawal
Poor Impulse Control
Insecure Attachment

The vagus nerve is the tenth of twelve paired cranial nerves, it extends through the jugular foramen, then passing into the carotid sheath between the internal carotid artery and the internal jugular vein down below the head, to the neck, chest and abdomen, where it contributes to the innervation of the viscera.

Besides output to the various organs in the body the vagus nerve conveys sensory information about the state of the body's organs to the central nervous system. 80-90% of the nerve fibres in the vagus nerve are afferent (sensory) nerves communicating the state of the viscera to the brain (Berthoud & Neuhuber, 2000). In the thorax branches go to the lungs for broncho-constriction, the oesophagus for peristalsis and the heart for slowing of heart rate. In the abdomen branches enter the stomach, pancreas, small intestine, large intestine and colon for secretion and constriction of smooth muscle.

The vagus nerve runs from the brain through the face and thorax to the abdomen. It is a mixed nerve that contains parasympathetic fibres. The vagus nerve has two sensory ganglia: the superior and the inferior ganglia. The branches of the superior ganglion innervate the skin in the concha of the ear. The inferior ganglion gives off two branches: the pharyngeal nerve and the superior laryngeal nerve.

The mammalian vagus is neuroanatomically linked to the cranial nerves that regulate social engagement via facial expression and vocalisation. The Polyvagal Theory provides neurobiological explanations for two dimensions of intimacy: courting and the establishment of enduring pair-bonds. The establishment of enduring pair-bonds is dependent upon a co-opting of the visceral vagus from an immobilisation system associated with fear and avoidance to a mobilisation system associated with safety and trust. The theory proposes that the phylogenetic development of the mammalian vagus is paralleled by a specialised communication, via oxytocin and vasopressin, between the hypothalamus and the medullary source nuclei of the visceral vagus.

The first stage is characterised by a primitive unmyelinated visceral vagus that fosters digestion and responds to threat by depressing metabolic activity. Behaviourally, the first stage is associated with immobilisation behaviours.

The second stage is characterised by the sympathetic nervous system that is capable of increasing metabolic output and inhibiting the visceral vagus to foster mobilisation behaviours necessary for 'fight or flight'.

The third stage, unique to mammals, is characterised by a myelinated vagus that can rapidly regulate cardiac output to foster engagement and disengagement with the environment (Porges, 1998).

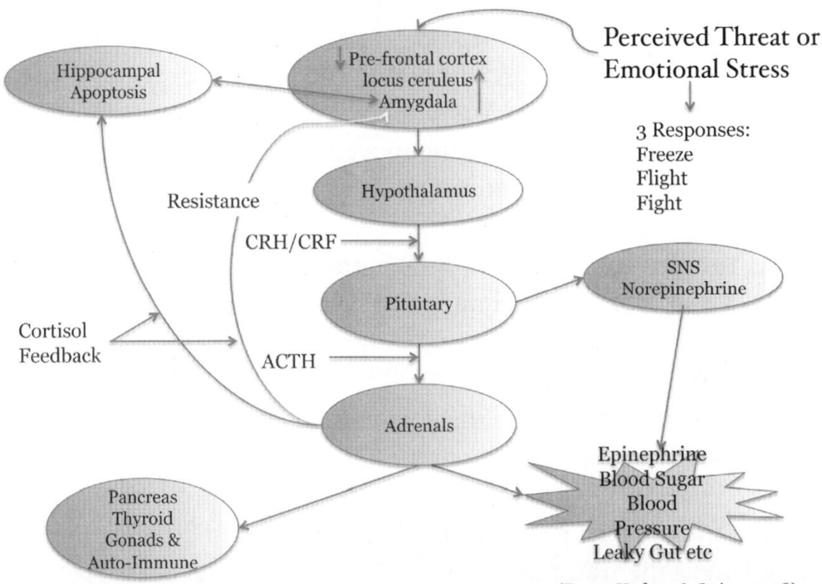

(From: Hedaya & Quinn 2008)[24]

The hypothalamus-pituitary-adrenal (HPA) axis prepares the body for challenge (stress). The feedback mechanism of the HPA Axis is designed to shut down its function when threat is finished. Excessive cortisol induces apoptosis (cell death) in the hippocampus.

San Jiao or Triple Energiser 三焦

The Zhong Zang Jing says: "The San Jiao is the leader of the five Zang and the six Fu, the Ying, the Wei and the Jingluo, the internal and external, the right and left, the upper and lower qi." The fundamental reason why the San Jiao possesses such an important position is that it controls the flow and motion of the Yuan qi (primordial qi). The Nan Jing says: "The life force that moves below the navel between the Kidneys, the root of the twelve channels, is by its old name called Yuan. The San Jiao is the transmitter of the Yuan qi, and it controls the movement of the three qi passing through the five Zang and six Fu".

The Yuan qi is the original moving force of the body, and is the root of the organs and channels. Through the San Jiao the Yuan qi reaches the entire body.

In the upper part it drives through the Heart and Lungs and nourishes and moves qi and blood.

In the middle part it penetrates the Stomach and Spleen and rots and ripens the water and grain.

In the lower part it pushes through the Liver and Kidney and dredges and reduces the bodily fluids (Lao, 1990).

Polyvagal Tone Theory

Stephen W. Porges' systematic investigation of mind-body relations has become the scientific basis for the science of psychophysiology. Unlike the correlative view of mind-body evaluations that dominates psychology and psychiatry, psychophysiology emphasises continuity between neuro-physiological and psychological processing. Psycho-physiologists assume that the nervous system provides the functional units for the bidirectional transduction of psychological and physiological processes. Thus, from a psychophysiological perspective, it is possible to link, not merely in theory, but also via measurement, psychological processes with neuro-physiological processes and brain structures (Porges, 1995). In simple terms the brain, gut and heart are linked and inseparable in the context of function; psyche and soma are one.

The evolution of the autonomic nervous system provides an organising principle to interpret the adaptive significance of physiological responses in promoting social behaviour. According to the Polyvagal theory, the well-documented phylogenetic shift in neural regulation of the autonomic nervous system passes through three global stages, each with an associated behavioural strategy.

The first stage is characterised by a primitive unmyelinated visceral vagus that fosters digestion and responds to threat by depressing metabolic activity. Behaviourally, the first stage is associated with immobilisation behaviours.

The second stage is characterised by the sympathetic nervous system that is capable of increasing metabolic output and inhibiting the visceral vagus to foster mobilisation behaviours necessary for 'fight or flight'.

The third stage, unique to mammals, is characterised by a myelinated vagus that can rapidly regulate cardiac output to foster engagement and disengagement with the environment (Porges, 1998). The implications of Porges's theory are both revolutionary from a Western point of view but confirming from a traditional medicine point of view. He says that part of the nervous system regulates our capacity to relate and to regulate our more fundamental flight/fight impulses. Our emotions are part of a network made up of physical function (body), perception (brain) and social network. Depression, anxiety, distress are all dysfunctions of this regulation system and have social (withdrawal/aggression), physical (obesity, heart disease, gut dysfunction) and perceptual (world view/attitude) implications. Medicines, which alter vagal tone will have whole being impact.

Polyvagal Tone: Psychophysiology

Psychophysiology emphasises continuity between neuro-physiological and psychological processing. Psycho-physiologists assume that the nervous system provides the functional units for the bi-directional transduction of psychological and physiological processes. Thus, from a psychophysiological perspective, it is possible to link psychological processes with neuro-physiological processes and brain structures (Porges, 1995).

The mammalian vagus is neuroanatomically linked to the cranial nerves that regulate social engagement via facial expression and vocalisation. As the autonomic nervous system changed through the process of evolution, so did the interplay between the autonomic nervous system and the other physiological systems that respond to stress, including the cortex, the HPA axis, the neuropeptides of oxytocin and vasopressin, and the immune system (Porges, 2001).

The evolution of the autonomic nervous system provides an organising principle to interpret the adaptive significance of mammalian affective processes including courting, sexual arousal, copulation, and the establishment of enduring social bonds.

The Polyvagal Theory provides neurobiological explanations for two dimensions of intimacy: courting and the establishment of enduring pair bonds.

Courting is dependent upon the social engagement strategies associated with the mammalian vagus. The establishment of enduring pair-bonds is dependent upon a co-opting of the visceral vagus from an immobilisation system associated with fear and avoidance to an immobilisation system associated with safety and trust (Porges, 1998).

The Polyvagal Theory demonstrates how issues of trust, love and cooperation arise when vagal tone is high and how it can suppress the other aspect of the ANS, the sympathetic nervous system (SNS). As a rule only one function or branch of the ANS can be dominant and high level of stress active SNS and suppress the vagus branch. The corresponding physical symptoms of SNS domination are just a pole to the emotional/cognitive issues, which may or may not be diagnosed.

Any intervention, which increases vagal tone and suppresses SNS activities, will alter both physical and psychological symptoms.

Chinese Herbal Medicine, Vagaltone and Triple Warmer 三焦

A clear correlation can be made between the affect of the vagal nerve and the function of the Triple Warmer (TW) in traditional Chinese medicine (TCM). This TCM model, is one of the oldest and simplest attempts to understand the workings of the body attempted by early Chinese medical scientists, references to it that can be found in the oldest medical texts available, including the Huang Di Nei Jing.

San Jiao has been translated as "triple heater," "triple warmer" (TW) (or three warmers), and "triple burner," the latter of which is probably favoured because of the involvement of the San Jiao in metabolism (burner meaning "metaboliser"). The current WHO standard term is "Triple Energiser" (TE).

The Shang Jiao [upper burner] - corresponding to the thoracic cavity. This space includes Fei [Lungs] and Xin [Heart].

The Zhong Jiao [middle burner] - corresponding to the upper part of the dorsal cavity. This space includes Wei [Stomach], Pi, usually called "Spleen", but better called the "nutrient uptake system". In WMS terminology, the Hepatic Portal System, various secretory pancreatic cells, perhaps the duodenum, portions of the lymphatic system carrying chyle, as well as catabolic and transaminioc functions of Liver cells and is associated with digestion.

The Xia Jiao [lower burner] - corresponding to the lower part of the dorsal cavity. This space includes Xiao Chang [small intestine], Da Chang [large intestine], Shen [Kidneys], Pang Guang

[Bladder] and is associated with elimination (West TCM, 2009). The San Jiao has no form, it is not an organ, and it is a collection of functions. The Classic of Difficulties says that the Yuan qi resides between the Kidneys and spreads to the Zang Fu via the San Jiao, it then enters the twelve meridians and emerges at the Yuan-source points. The Yuan qi can only make possible all body functions through its spreading by the San Jiao. Therefore it greatly effects the warming for digestion, and excretion (ibid).

The qi of the "triple origin" of man has great impact on the whole of the Zang Fu and "When the triple heater ensures free communication, then there is free communication internally and externally, left and right, above and below. The whole body is irrigated, harmonised internally and regulated externally, nourished by the left, and maintained by the right, directed from above, propagated from below. There is nothing greater!" Hua Tuo (Larre and Vallee, 1992). The TW is an organ system that has no 'physical' presence but could clearly relate to those aspects of the ANS, which control heart rate and blood pressure, gastric and duodenal function and bowel function. The TW is a transformative organ. The complexity of vagal tone, enteric nervous and endocrine systems and their relationship to the CNS is critical in treating Shen disorders.

Shen
神

Although the etymological origin of shen is uncertain, Schuessler (2007) notes a possible Sino-Tibetan etymology; comparing it to Chepang gliŋh or "spirit of humans". The primary meaning of shen is translatable as "spirit, spirits, Spirit, spiritual beings;

celestial spirits; ancestral spirits" or "god, gods, God; deity, deities, supernatural beings", etc. Shen is sometimes loosely translated as "soul", but Chinese medicine distinguishes hun 魂 "spiritual soul" and po 魄 "physical soul" (Mateer, 1901).

Paleographers interpret the Oracle script of 申 as a pictograph of a "lightning bolt" semantically suggesting both "lightning" and "spirits" coming down from the heavens, also 'to speak' (Schuessler, 2007). The origin of the first part of the character in Shen 神 has been identified as shi 示, which is the sun arises above the sea with reflection. Shen could be interpreted as 'radiance speaking'. Shen is a function of positivity, consciousness, communication and stability. Shen personifies the fiery spark of conscious awareness. During our life, the shen is said to reside in the empty centre of the heart from where it guides us along our path through life.

Qi
氣

The etymological explanation for the form of the qi logogram in the traditional form 氣 is "steam (气) rising from rice (米) as it cooks. Another, more pertinent way of seeing qi is that of transformation. The changing of form in which a material substance is converted to energy, that is qi is not a thing but a process. It is the capacity to change.

"There is but one qi all under the heaven." "When man is born, his qi is gathered. When his qi is gathered, his life thrives. When his qi is dispersed, his life dies out" (Guo, 1997).

Qi comes to embrace properties, which we would call psychic, emotional, spiritual, numinous, and even 'mystic' (Schwartz, 1985). The concept of qi then is the primal energy underlying all matter, moulded as cloud vapour and breath. It gives life to living beings. Qi gives us vitality, and the vital energy of the heart/mind, which controls our thoughts and emotions, and moral sensibilities and our body and physical activities (Gao, 1996).

According to Confucius, qi is the source of emotional behaviour: "In youth, one's blood and qi are not yet settled, one guards against lust. Having reached maturity, one's blood and qi is firm, one guards against aggressiveness. Having reached old age, one's blood and qi are in decline, one guards against avarice" (The Analects). Qi transformation encompasses all the functional activities of qi in the body, including blood circulation, essence transformation, body fluid movement, waste excretion, skin moistening, nutrient absorption, sinew and bone moistening, and resistance.

Herbs can affect most of the above activities, the vagus nerve may be involved in their functions, but there may be more underlying or complicated mechanisms. Chinese herbal medicinals clearly have an impact on the vagus nerve and, speculatively an affect on mood, stress and cognitive function.

CHINESE MEDICINE PATTERNS

Blood Circulation

As early as the Warring States period (475-221) a major work of medicine appeared in China: *The Classic of Internal Medicine*, consisting of two books: *Plain Questions* and the *Miraculous Pivot*. These books introduced the idea that the heart is the centre of blood circulation and of the system of blood vessels of the human body and that the blood circulating in the vessels "is similar to a flow of water, travelling around without end". The main function of 'blood' is to nourish and moisten the body.

Blood Stagnation

When the flow of Blood is blocked or stagnated it means the Blood is not flowing freely. An injury or a blockage of energy circulation can cause this.

The primary symptom of Blood Stagnation is pain; the sensation of this pain is deep, fixed and stabbing in nature. The most frequent types of pain resulting from blood stasis are pain in the lower abdomen, chest pain, pain from trauma and pain as a result of internal bleeding. There may also be a dark complexion, delayed menses and purplish nails. Diseases caused by Blood Stagnation or impeded Blood Circulation include abdominal masses, delayed menses with dark blood and blood clots, amenorrhoea, (no menses) postpartum abdominal pain, trauma, rheumatic pain, carbuncles and ulcers. Dark, purple tongue, may have purple spots. Thready, uneven pulse.

Blood Deficiency

If the 'blood' becomes deficient, the body will lack nourishment. The cause of 'blood deficiency' may be:

1. Massive loss of blood
2. Decreased ability of the spleen and stomach to transform food essence into blood and
3. Internal damage to 'blood' due to protracted illness; this will lead to symptoms of weakness. There may be dizziness, dry eyes, blurred

, pale complexion, palpitations, shortness of breath, numbness of hands and feet, delayed menstruation or amenorrhea, stiff joints. Pale Tongue and thready or feeble pulse.

The main function of 'blood' is to nourish and moisten the body, ensuring the body tissues do not dry out. Blood deficiency simply means that the blood is not nourishing the body as it should. "Blood' has also a functional relationship with the Mind providing a stable foundation. If 'Blood is deficient, the Mind will be unhappy or uneasy with such symptoms as vague anxiety, mild irritability and a sense of dissatisfaction. General signs for Blood deficiency may be dizziness, blurred vision, pale complexion, dry skin and hair loss and there may be menstrual problems.
Symptoms: pale or sallow complexion, pale lips and fingernails, blurred vision, dizziness, palpitations and insomnia, numbness of hands and feet, rough skin, delayed menstruation or amenorrhoea. Tongue pale. Pulse empty.

Blood Cold
Symptoms: Coldness and pain in the hands and feet as well as lower abdomen, which can be relieved by warmth. Aversion to cold, preference for warmth, irregular menstrual cycle, dysmenorrhoea—painful menstrual cycle, dark purple menses with clots. Tongue pale with white coating. Pulse slow and deep.

Blood Heat
Symptoms: shortened menstrual cycle, menorrhagia - excessive menstrual flow. Any bleeding patterns - from eyes, ears, nose, mouth,

haemoptysis, excessive thirst. Tongue red. Pulse slippery, rapid.

Dampness Pathogenic Influence causing Stagnation in the Spleen and Stomach

Dampness can be either cold-dampness or damp-heat. The spleen dislikes dampness and dampness retained in the middle jiao impairs the function of the spleen and stomach. Aromatic herbs dispel dampness, activate the circulation of qi and strengthen spleen and gastric function. The primary manifestations of this process are a feeling of distension and fullness in the chest and abdomen, nausea, vomiting, anorexia, heaviness of the head and body, lack of thirst, reduced appetite, heavy feeling in the limbs, sticky and greasy taste in the mouth, excessive saliva, diarrhoea with some difficulty in defecation, urinary turbidity, and a soggy pulse with a thick greasy tongue coating.

Dampness as damp-heat refers to disorders with Heat signs, fever, burning sensations, and dark, yellow secretions together with retention of Dampness. Symptoms include painful urination, purulent rashes and jaundice. Damp-heat can also refer to obstructions in the respiratory and digestive systems; this may include phlegm retention in chronic bronchitis and water retention in the stomach due to gastritis.

Dampness Draining

Draining dampness involves increasing the urine production, as this is the primary way in which Dampness is relieved. Dampness is mainly caused by dysfunction of the Bladder or Yang Deficiency of the Spleen and Kidneys resulting in failure to regulate the flow of Qi and water, also for water accumulation in the body or for various disorders caused by the combination of dampness with heat or cold pathogenic factors. Indications for Dampness are water and dampness retention, dysuria, oedema, ascites, phlegm retention, stranguria, jaundice and dampness-warm syndrome. In modern medical terms, herbs used to drain dampness are primarily diuretics.

Disturbances of the Spirit

Clearly one of the most useful points in Chinese Medicine is its recognition of the psychospiritual aspects of the person and how these manifest physically. In our everyday hectic life the Spirit can easily be affected and as a result manifests anxiety, stress, insomnia or palpitations. Disorders of the spirit are either of deficiency or of the excess type. The former symptoms belong to the Deficiency type whereas the excess type of disturbance of the spirit includes being overstressed, manic behaviour, bad temper and agitation.

Food Stagnation

Food Stagnation is mainly Hot or Cold. Symptoms of Hot Food Stagnation are severe bad breath, abdominal distension, aversion to hot food and drink and a preference for cold ones, a yellow greasy tongue coating and a strong slippery pulse. Cold Food Stagnation arises from Stomach or Spleen Deficiency or overindulgence in cold food. Symptoms are nausea, spitting up clear fluids, abdominal distension, preference for hot food and drink and aversion to cold ones, a tongue with a white greasy coating and a weak, thin pulse.

Heat Syndromes

Heat syndromes are categorised as being exterior or interior heat, and excess or deficiency heat. There are four major categories.

Internal Heat & Fire

Two sub categories are, a) internal heat from exogenous pathogenic factors: - excess heat in the qi system marked by persistent high fever (as in febrile diseases - restlessness and thirst) and b) endogenous or internal fire in the organs. Symptoms are dependent on the organ system most affected.

Lung heat may manifest as sore throat cough, shortness of breath, wheezing, dryness, may or may not have skin rash. Heart heat may manifest as fever, thirst dry mouth, restlessness irritability and possible insomnia. A stomach heat syndrome may present as sever thirst, dry mouth, hunger, halitosis, and desire for cold drinks. Liver heat may manifest in ophthalmic symptoms i.e. dry red painful eyes and or blurred vision, irritability, hypochondriac pain and distension, menstrual changes may occur in female patients – changes in cycle and flow. Kidney heat may present as night sweating, low-grade fever or less commonly, bleeding gums.

Toxic Heat

This pattern is usually seen in the later stage of externally contracted diseases. Main Symptoms: high fever, irascibility and thirst, skin eruptions and in extreme expression of mania hematemesis and melaena.

Blood Heat

Clinical manifestations of blood heat include hemoptysis, or hematemesis, bleeding, hematuria, hematochezia, advanced profuse menstruation, even åmetrorrhagia, dysphoria, thirst, deep reddish tongue and fast pulse.

Deficiency Heat

Deficiency heat due to yin deficiency, late stage febrile diseases leading to fever during the night and chills in the morning. Symptoms: gradual onset, long duration; fluctuant low-grade, spontaneous sweating, dry mouth, shortness breath and general weakness. The pulse is thready and rapid; the tongue is red with little fur.

Interior Cold Syndrome

Interior cold patterns can be classified into two categories: the first one is cold invasion into the spleen and stomach which creates hypofunction of the digestive system with such symptoms as gastric and abdominal pain, nausea, vomiting, belching and diarrhoea; the second one is cold internally generated as a result of deficiency of yang-qi. Symptoms in mild cases of internally generated Cold deficiency patterns include aversion to cold, cold extremities, pallid complexion, loose stool, lack of thirst with desire for hot liquids, loose stools, thin white tongue coating and a slow pulse.

Kidney Essence
Deficiency of Kidney Essence is involved with slow development and maturity. Bones do not develop properly, there is premature ageing, problems with the menstrual cycle and sometimes with conception as seen in infertility in men due to low sperm count and in women due to amenorrhoea, genitals may fail to develop properly, birth defects. There may be premature greying of the hair, or balding, also loosened teeth. There may be congenital retardation and many other genetic disorders, as well as impotence and low libido.

Kidney Yang Deficiency
Symptoms: aversion to cold, cold hands and feet, soreness and pain in the lower back and knees, increased urination at night, impotence, seminal emission, premature ejaculation, leukorrhea, dizziness, ringing in the ears. Pale, swollen tongue with white coating, deep and thready pulse.

Kidney Yin Deficiency
Symptoms: Weakness in the loins and knees, dizziness, tinnitus, insomnia, hot hands, feet and heart area, afternoon fever, malar flush, night sweats, nocturnal emission, scanty menstruation, amenorrhoea, uterine bleeding. Red tongue with little coating, rapid pulse.

Liver Patterns

Liver invading the Spleen
The liver is responsible for the smooth flow of energy through the system and can therefore directly affect other organs; the spleen's

primary function concerns digestion and transformation of foods. The Spleen assimilates nutrients from the food, which is then sent throughout the body. The smooth flow of energy helps to regulate emotional activities, thus preventing depression or moodiness. When the Spleen is weakened usually through dietary habits, the Liver may overwhelm the spleen. Some of the symptoms of this syndrome are alternating constipation and diarrhoea, tiredness, irritability, abdominal distension and fullness in the chest. The tongue may be pale, or red on the sides.

Liver Blood Deficiency

As well as being responsible for the smooth flow of qi, the liver stores blood. When liver blood becomes deficient a number of symptoms may arise: dizziness, dry eyes, blurred vision, tinnitus, anaemia, night blindness, spasm of the tendons, numbness of the limbs, pale or brittle nails, trembling hands and feet and in women scanty menstrual flow or amenorrhoea, pale tongue with white coating and a fine pulse.

Liver Qi Stagnation

When the Liver Qi is stagnant, the energy does not flow freely which give rise to emotional disturbances. The reverse is also possible, if there is emotional repression, the liver qi will in time become stagnant. Liver Qi stagnation generally results in irritability, anger, depression, frequent sighing, painful menstruation, irregular periods, pain under the ribs, loss of appetite and any symptoms that get worse with emotional turmoil.

Liver Yang Rising

Main symptoms: Dizziness, flushed face, tinnitus, distending pain in the head and the eyes, red eyes, heavy feeling in the head, insomnia, palpitations. Red tongue, taut and rapid pulse.

Liver Yin Deficiency

Dry eyes are a symptom of Liver Yin Deficiency, as the yin of the liver is unable to moisten the eyes. Other symptoms are dizziness, tinnitus, blurred vision, hot feeling in hands and feet, night sweats. Tongue is red and the pulse is rapid and thready.

Lung Patterns

While Western medicine ascribes to the lungs the primary task of respiration, Chinese medicine adds the function of qi circulation. Furthermore Chinese medicine adds that the Lungs govern healthy functioning of hair and skin. The Lungs play an essential role in controlling the blood vessels and also regulates the dispersing of qi to keep the Water passages unobstructed.

Lung Qi Deficiency

Symptoms: spontaneous sweating, feeble cough that is worse on exertion, a propensity to catch frequent colds, weak cough, fatigue, light wheezing, shortness of breath, exhaustion, weak, low voice, watery sputum, lack of vitality, aversion to cold. Tongue red with yellow coating. Slippery, rapid pulse.

Lung Yin Deficiency

Symptoms: Dry cough or cough with sticky blood stained sputum, dry mouth and throat, flushed face and fever in the afternoon, night sweats, feverish sensation in the palms, soles and heart region. Tongue red with little coating. Pulse thready and rapid.

Lung Heat

Symptoms: Asthmatic cough, coarse breathing, thick, yellow sputum or cough with foul blood stained purulent sputum, fever, thirst, chest pain, sore throat, dry stool and deep-coloured scanty urine. Tongue red with yellow coating. Pulse slippery and rapid.

Phlegm Accumulation

Phlegm accumulation refers to the accumulation of fluids in the body cavity and extremities. Pathogenic phlegm can accumulate in the internal organs or in the tendons, bones, skin and muscles. Symptoms: Phlegm in the heart and/or heart channel: dementia, mental confusion, anxiety, a feeling of oppression in the chest, nausea, a feeling of heaviness and a 'fuzzy' head with dizziness. Tongue with swollen body with a sticky coating. Pulse slippery or wiry.

Purgatives
Purgatives are divided into three categories:

1. ***Potent Purgatives*** (*gong xia yao*) that are mostly bitter and cold and powerfully promotes bowel movement and purges heat. Used for retention of excess heat in the intestines. This could manifest as constipation, initial stages of dysentery due to heat in the large intestine, excess fire creating headache, red eyes, swelling and pain of the gums.
2. ***Lubricant Purgatives*** (*run xiao yao*), these herbs are sweet and mild and moisten and lubricate the bowels. They are mostly indicated for constipation as a result of intestinal dryness.
3. ***Drastic Purgatives*** (*jun xia zhu shui yao*) are mostly bitter, cold, toxic and drastic in their action, and can cause copious watery discharge. They can also have a diuretic effect, relieving fluid retention through urination and bowel movement and are indicated for oedema, fluid in the lungs and ascites.

Qi Patterns
Qi is a term that refers to our body's vital energy. It is what activates the growth and development of the human body, promotes the physiological functions of each viscous, bowel, channel, collateral, tissue and organ and speeds up the formation and circulation of blood and the metabolism of body fluid as well.

Qi Deficiency
Qi can easily become deficient, it is common in chronic conditions, during stages of recovery from acute conditions or simply due to our lifestyle, whether it is simply too demanding or stress-

ful. Symptoms: Not enough strength to breathe, or to speak, general weariness, dizziness, spontaneous sweating, listlessness with symptoms that get worse after exertion. Tongue pale and tender. Pulse weak.

Sinking of Qi

Sinking of qi is a symptom-complex in which qi-deficiency occurs. This is seen in the inability of the tissues to support due to the weakness of qi. Symptoms: prolapse of internal organs, stomach, kidney or uterus.

Stagnation of Qi

Qi stagnation is characterised by the blockage of qi in certain parts of the body or in a specific organ. This blockage impedes the flow of qi creating disorders such as endocrine disturbances, premenstrual tension. Symptoms: irritability, oppression and pain in the chest, hypochondrium and abdomen, frequent sighing, onset of pain or symptoms are related to emotions. Symptoms may be relieved by borborygmus or flatus. Exercise is helpful. Stagnation of qi is a symptom complex characterised by the blockage of qi in a certain part of the body or in an individual organ. When qi does not flow properly, distension and pain is the result.

Stagnant qi can be divided into three major types:

1. *Stagnant Spleen and Stomach qi* stagnation causing distending pain in the stomach and abdomen, poor appetite, belching, acid regurgitation, nausea, vomiting and diarrhoea or constipation. Adverse rise of Stomach qi is marked by nausea, vomiting, belching and hiccups.
2. *Liver qi Stagnation* with as primary symptoms distending pain in the chest, loss of appetite, depression, irritability and hernial pain. In women stagnant Liver qi may cause irregular menstruation and pain in the breasts.

3. *Lung qi Stagnation* which causes wheezing and cough with laboured breezing and distress in the chest.

Rebellious Qi

Rebellious qi indicates a disturbance in the upward or downward functions of the body. Symptoms: cough, belching, hiccups, nausea, vomiting, headache, dizziness.

Qi and Blood Deficiency

Symptoms: shortness of breath, reluctance to speak, listlessness, fatigue, vertigo, blurred vision, spontaneous perspiration, pale or sallow complexion, palpitations and insomnia. Tongue pale and flabby. Pulse thready and feeble.

Qi Regulation

Qi regulation deals with two disorders of qi: qi deficiency and qi stagnation. Deficiency of qi is a symptom complex in which there is hypo-functioning of the organs or of an individual organ; this is seen in chronic conditions, during recovery from acute diseases and during general recovery by old, weak patients.

Spleen Disharmony

The Spleen is primarily concerned with digestion and through this function it has a direct relationship with our energy. Spleen disharmony is often the result of poor dietary habits. Any Spleen disharmony will always involve the digestive process with such general symptoms as abdominal distension, loose stool and lack of appetite. Other symptoms might be weakness of the limbs, tiredness and abdominal pain. The tongue may be swollen and wet.

Spleen Qi Deficiency

Symptoms: Poor appetite, fullness in the abdomen after eating, fatigue, loose stools, pale or sallow complexion. Tongue with white coating. Pulse slow and weak.

Spleen Yang Deficiency

Symptoms: Poor appetite, abdominal distension, chills, cold limbs. Dull abdominal pain relieved by pressure and heat. Tongue pale with white coating. Pulse deep and feeble.

Damp-heat in the Spleen

Symptoms: Nausea, poor appetite, heavy sensation in limbs, sticky bitter taste in the mouth, feeling hot, loose stools, burning sensation when defecating, difficult urination with reddish tinge. Tongue red with yellow slimy coating. Pulse soft and rapid.

Stomach Yin Deficiency

Deficient Stomach Yin accounts for a lack of fluids in the stomach, which often occurs after serious febrile disorders. Symptoms: dull stomach-ache, gastric discomfort with acid regurgitation, hungry but not being able to eat, irritability, dry mouth and throat, constipation fullness in the upper abdomen, hiccups. Tongue red with little coating. Pulse thready and rapid.

Deficiency Syndromes of the Heart

Heart Blood Deficiency

General symptoms are dream disturbed sleep, palpitations, forgetfulness, insomnia and the signs are sallow complexion, dizziness, pale lips and tongue and a fine, thready pulse.

Heart Qi Deficiency

General symptoms are palpitations, shortness of breath, spontaneous sweating that is worse when active with as chief symptoms pale complexion, listlessness and fatigue, pale tongue with thin white coating, fine, weak, or irregular intermittent pulse.

Heart Yang Deficiency

Symptoms: bright, pale complexion, aversion to cold, cold limbs, oedema of hands and feet, cardiac retardation, fullness in the chest, purplish lips, pale and swollen tongue with white moist coating, thready, feeble pulse.

Heart Yin Deficiency

General symptoms are dream disturbed sleep, palpitations, insomnia, irritability, hot sensation in the palms and the soles, afternoon fever, night sweats, dry mouth and throat, tongue sores. Deep red and dry tongue. Thready, rapid pulse.

Excess Syndromes of the Heart

Flaring up of Heart Fire

Symptoms: Mouth and tongue ulcers, swollen and painful tongue, restlessness, insomnia, dry mouth, dark yellow urine, red tongue tip, rapid pulse.

Stagnation of Heart Blood and Obstruction of the Vessels

Symptoms: palpitations, sudden fullness or stabbing pain in the heart and chest, cold limbs, sweating, purplish lips and nails. Dark red tongue or tongue with purple spots. Choppy pulse.

Mental disturbance Due to Phlegm and Fire

Symptoms: uncontrolled emotions, severe anxiety or phobia, dream disturbed sleep, mental disorders, in severe cases mania. Red tongue with yellow slimy coating. Taut, slippery and strong pulse.

Obstruction of the Heart Channel by Phlegm

Symptoms: disturbance of the spirit, delirium, mania, coma, sound of phlegm in the throat. Tongue coating with white slimy phlegm. Pulse slippery.

Wind Dampness

Externally contracted Wind-dampness is generally a condition of excess. Wind dampness is marked by pain or sometimes numbness. This syndrome is also known as Bi-Syndrome, or painful obstruction. Bi syndromes tend to be caused by wind, cold and damp pathogenic factors blocking the channels, or by the obstruction of qi and Blood: main symptoms pain in the limbs and joints. The condition is characterised by a dull and heavy pain and numbness that can persist in certain joints, the nature and location of which depends on the depth of penetration of the pathogens and whether or not cold or heat is present. Rheumatic pain that gets worse in damp weather is a good example of this type of imbalance. Symptoms may also include a heavy feeling in the body or 'fuzzy' feeling in the head. Could also be loss of appetite, loose stools, sticky taste or vaginal discharge. The tongue may be swollen with a greasy coat and the pulse will be slippery.

Yang Deficiency

The bodies' Yang is associated with warming, movement and energy. A deficiency of yang means the heat of the body has been damaged and this will result in too much cold internally. Signs of yang deficiency will be loose stools, cold hands and feet and a pale complexion. Symptoms: Listlessness, lassitude, desire to curl up, apathy, weak voice, chills, cold limbs, spontaneous sweating, absence of thirst, clear urine with increased volume, loose stools. Tongue pale with white coating. Pulse weak.

Yin Deficiency

The bodies' Yin energy is associated with moistening, cooling and nourishing. Deficient yin indicates the fluids of the body have been damaged which will result in symptoms of heat. Some signs associated with yin deficiency will be night sweats, hot flushes, thirst, and a red flushed face. Symptoms: afternoon fever, malar flush, feverish sensation in the palms, soles and heart region, night sweats, dryness of mouth and throat, yellow urine and dry stools. Tongue red with little coating. Pulse thready and rapid.

CHINESE HERBAL MEDICINE AND VAGUS NERVE

1. Superficial-Syndrome Relieving

Herb Name	Pharmaceutical Functions	
	Organ Function	**Descriptions**
ma huang Ephedra sinica	Sweat Gland	Significantly excites sweat gland, promotes perspiration
	Smooth Muscle	Relaxes and relieves the smooth muscle of the bronchi Relaxes the smooth muscle of gastrointestinal muscle Inhibits gastrointestinal peristalsis
xi xin Asarum heterothropoides	Smooth Muscle	Increases and then reduces the tension of isolated intestinal canals in rabbits; takes on an inhibitory effect at high concentrations Relaxes ileac spasm induced by histamine, acetylcholine and BaCl2
jing jie Schizonepeta tenuifolia	Respiratory System	Relaxes isolated bronchi in animals
	Digestive System	Takes on an inhibitory effect on the duodenal smooth muscle
fang feng Saposhnikovia divaricata	Digestive System	Significantly reduces the contraction of smooth muscle in isolated intestines
	Cardiovascular System	Lowers blood pressure

<table>
<tr><th rowspan="2">Herb Name</th><th colspan="2">Pharmaceutical Functions</th></tr>
<tr><th>Organ Function</th><th>Descriptions</th></tr>
<tr><td rowspan="2">sheng jiang
Zingiber
officinale</td><td>Digestive System</td><td>Anti-ulcerative
Antiemetic
Increases secretions of gastric juice
Relaxes the smooth muscles of intestinal canals
Inhibits the contraction of stomach in situ
Promotes bile secretions</td></tr>
<tr><td>Cardio-vascular System</td><td>Lowers blood pressure and reduces heart rate transitorily</td></tr>
<tr><td rowspan="2">zi su
Perilla
frutescens</td><td>Digestive System</td><td>Promotes secretions of digestive juices
Promotes gastrointestinal peristalsis</td></tr>
<tr><td>Respiratory System</td><td>Relieves bronchial spasm</td></tr>
<tr><td rowspan="2">bai zhi
Angelica
dahurica</td><td>Cardio-vascular System</td><td>Dilates coronary vessel
Different ingredients have different actions (dilation or contraction) on vessels</td></tr>
<tr><td>Smooth Muscle</td><td>Inhibits spontaneous movements of isolated small intestines</td></tr>
<tr><td rowspan="3">gao ben
Ligusticum
sinense</td><td>Smooth Muscle</td><td>Inhibits smooth muscles of intestines</td></tr>
<tr><td>Cardio-vascular System</td><td>Lowers blood pressure</td></tr>
<tr><td>Lowers blood pressure</td><td>Antiasthmatic, relieves spasms of smooth muscles</td></tr>
<tr><td>xiang ru
Elsholtzia
splendens</td><td>Smooth Muscle</td><td>Significantly inhibits spontaneous contraction of isolated ileum</td></tr>
</table>

Herb Name	Pharmaceutical Functions	
	Organ Function	**Descriptions**
xin yi Magnolia liliflora	Cardio-vascular System	Dilates blood vessels Lowers blood pressure
	Respiratory System	Excites respiration
cang er zi Xanthium sibiricum	Cardio-vascular System	Inhibits isolated hearts Reduces heart rate and contractile force Lowers blood pressure temporarily
	Respiratory System	Excites respiration at small dosages while inhibits respiration at large dosages
e bu shi cao Centipeda minima	Respiratory System	Antiasthmatic
ding gong teng Erycibe obtusfolia	Cardio-vascular System	Significantly reduces heart rate Significantly increases myocardial contractive Lowers oxygen consumption of cardiac muscle
	Smooth Muscle	Significantly inhibits contraction of isolated ileum
chai hu Bupleurum chinense	Digestive System	Significantly inhibits secretions of gastric juice, increases ph value of gastric contents; lowers pepsin activity and ulcerative index Excites isolated intestines Promotes bile output
ge gen Pueraria lobata	Cardio-vascular System	Reduces heart rate and cardiac output Dilates blood vessels Lowers blood pressure
	Smooth Muscle	Different ingredients have different functions (excitatory and inhibitory) on intestines

<table>
<tr><th rowspan="2">Herb Name</th><th colspan="2">Pharmaceutical Functions</th></tr>
<tr><th>Organ Function</th><th>Descriptions</th></tr>
<tr><td rowspan="2">sheng ma
Cimicifuga dahurica</td><td>Cardio-vascular System</td><td>Inhibits the heart
Reduces heart rate
Lowers blood pressure</td></tr>
<tr><td>Smooth Muscle</td><td>Relieves spasms of intestinal smooth muscle</td></tr>
<tr><td>ju hua
Chrysanthe-mum morifolium</td><td>Cardio-vascular System</td><td>Significantly dilates isolated coronary blood vessels
Increases blood flow volume in coronary blood vessels
Reduces heart rate</td></tr>
<tr><td>bo he
Mentha haplocalyx</td><td>Digestive System</td><td>Menthol and menthone inhibits movements and relieves spasms of intestinal movements
Increases bile secretions</td></tr>
<tr><td rowspan="2">sang ye
Morus alba</td><td>Smooth Muscle</td><td>Inhibits intestinal muscles</td></tr>
<tr><td>Cardio-vascular System</td><td>Temporarily lowers blood pressure</td></tr>
<tr><td rowspan="2">niu bang zi
Arctium lappa</td><td>Cardio-vascular System</td><td>Anaesthetises isolated heart
Persistently lowers blood pressure</td></tr>
<tr><td>Smooth Muscle</td><td>Inhibits or anaesthetised isolated intestines</td></tr>
<tr><td rowspan="2">mu zei
Equisetum hyemale</td><td>Cardio-vascular System</td><td>Dilates blood vessels
Lowers blood pressure</td></tr>
<tr><td>Digestive System</td><td>Extracts at different concentration have different functions
(inhibitory or excitatory)
on isolated intestines or ileum</td></tr>
<tr><td>man jing zi
Vitex rotundifolia</td><td>Cardio-vascular System</td><td>Lowers blood pressure</td></tr>
</table>

2. Heat Clearing

Herb Name	Pharmaceutical Functions	
	Organ Function	Descriptions
jin yin hua Lonicera japonica	Digestive System	Chlorogenic acid promotes bile secretions
da qing ye Isatis tinctoria	Digestive System	Inhibits isolated intestines
	Cardio-vascular System	Inhibits isolated heart
pu gong ying Taraxacum mongolicum	Digestive System	Promotes bile secretions Increases tension of isolated duodenum
shan dou gen Sophora subprostrata	Digestive System	Relieves intestinal spasms Anti-ulcerative, inhibits secretions of gastric juice
bei dou gen Menisper-mum dauricum	Cardio-vascular System	Lowers blood pressure
	Digestive System	Inhibits secretions of gastric juice Significantly inhibits isolated or in situ small intestines and relieves spasms
chuan xin lian Andrographis paniculata	Digestive System	Promotes bile secretions
zhong jie feng Sarcandra glaba	Digestive System	Anti-ulcerative, inhibits secretions of gastric juice
yu xing cao Houttuynia cordata	Respiratory System	Antiasthmatic, relieves isolated bronchial smooth muscle
	Cardio-vascular System	Lowers blood pressure
qin pi Fraxinus rhynchophylla	Digestive System	Inhibits isolated intestinal muscles
	Respiratory System	Antiasthmatic, relaxes smooth muscles of isolated tracheae

Herb Name	Pharmaceutical Functions	
	Organ Function	**Descriptions**
ye ju hua Chrysanthemum indicum	Cardiovascular System	Lowers blood pressure
	Digestive System	Relieves spasms of isolated small intestine
bai xian pi Dictamnus dasycarpus	Digestive System	Inhibits contraction of small intestine Relaxes Oddi's sphincter
shi gao Gypsum fibrosum	Digestive System	Bi-directional actions on isolated small intestines: small dosages increases amplitude while large dosages lowers its tension and amplitude
zhi zi Gardenia jasminoides	Digestive System	Contracts gallbladder and increases bile secretions Increases tension of isolated intestinal canal and decreases its peristalsis Decreases secretions of gastric juice
	Cardiovascular System	Significantly inhibits heart in situ Reduces blood pressure and lowers heart rate simultaneously
xia ku cao Prunella vulgaris	Cardiovascular System	Lowers blood pressure
lian xin Plumula nelumbinis nuciferae	Cardiovascular System	Lowers blood pressure
huang qin Scutellaria baicalensis	Cardiovascular System	Lowers blood pressure
huang lian Coptis chinensis	Cardiovascular System	Reduces heart rate slowly but persistently after a reactive increase Increases myocardial contractive Lowers blood pressure
huang bo Phellodendron amurense	Digestive System	Anti-ulcerative Significantly inhibits gastric juice, total acidity, and total pepsin activity

Herb Name	Pharmaceutical Functions	
	Organ Function	Descriptions
huang bo Phelloden-dron amu-rense	Cardio-vascular System	Lowers blood pressure
long dan cao Gentiana scabra	Digestive System	Increases bile flow
shui niu jiao Cornu bubali	Cardio-vascular System	Lowers blood pressure
	Digestive System	Increases tension and movements of isolated intestinal canal
xuan shen Scrophularia ningpoensis	Cardio-vascular System	Lowers blood pressure Slightly inhibits heart rate, myocardial contractive
mu dan pi Paeonia suffruticosa	Cardio-vascular System	Reduces heart rate
chi shao Paeonia lactiflora	Cardio-vascular System	Lowers pulmonary artery pressure
	Smooth Muscle	Lowers tension of isolated duodenum Antagonises gastric contraction caused by pilocarpine
zi cao Lithosper-mum erythro-rhizon	Cardio-vascular System	Increases myocardial contractive Reduces blood pressure dramatically and transitorily
qing hao Artemisia annua	Cardio-vascular System	Reduces heart rate and myocardial contractive Lowers blood flow of coronary vessels Reduces blood pressure
di gu pi Lycium chinense	Cardio-vascular System	Reduces heart rate
hu huang lian Picrorhiza scrophulariaeflora	Digestive System	Increases bile flow

3. Purgatives

Herb Name	Pharmaceutical Functions	
	Organ Function	**Descriptions**
da huang Rheum palmatum	Digestive System	Promotes bile secretions Anti-ulcerative Lowers volume of gastric juice, free acid in gastric juice and pepsin activity
	Smooth Muscle	Excites electric activity of colon
fan xie ye Cassia angustifolia	Smooth Muscle	Increases amplitude of ileac movements Antagonises spasmodic contraction of ileum induced by acetylcholine
huo ma ren Cannabis sativa	Cardio-vascular System	Lowers blood pressure
qian niu zi Pharbitis purpurea	Smooth Muscle	Excites smooth muscles of small and large intestines
ba dou Croton tiglium	Digestive System	Promotes gastrointestinal peristalsis

4. Wind-Dampness Eliminating

Herb Name	Pharmaceutical Functions	
	Organ Function	**Descriptions**
qin jiao Gentiana macrophylla	Cardio-vascular System	Lowers blood pressure Reduces heart rate
wei lin xian Clematis chinensis	Smooth Muscle	Relaxes sphincter at the end of common bile duct
	Cardio-vascular System	Significantly lowers blood pressure

Herb Name	Pharmaceutical Functions	
	Organ Function	**Descriptions**
fen fang ji Stephania tetrandra	Smooth Muscle	Excites intestines in situ Increases tension of isolated intestines and increases its rhythmic contraction at low dosages, takes on contrary functions at high dosages Relaxes isolated bronchial smooth muscle at low dosages, while contracts it at high dosages
	Cardio-vascular System	Significantly lowers contraction of cardiac muscle Significantly lowers heart rate Reduces heart rate Dilates coronary blood vessel, lowers blood flow volume in kidneys, spleen, mesentery and portal vein
xi xian cao Siegesbeckia orientalis	Cardio-vascular System	Lowers blood pressure
chuan wu Aconitum carmichaeli	Cardio-vascular System	Dilates blood vessels Lowers blood pressure Cardiac tonic
ma qian zi Strychnos pierriana	Digestive System	Increases secretions of gastric juice
sang ji sheng Viscum coloratum	Cardio-vascular System	Lowers blood pressure Dilates coronary blood vessels Reduces heart rate
hai feng teng Piper futokadsura	Cardio-vascular System	Dilates coronary vessels

Herb Name	Pharmaceutical Functions	
	Organ Function	Descriptions
qing feng teng Sinomenium acutum	Cardio-vascular System	Lowers blood pressure
	Digestive System	Lowers tension of isolated ileum Inhibits intestinal muscle contraction induced by pilocarpine, histamine Increases secretions of gastric juice and total acidity
lu xian cao Pyrola rotundifolia	Cardio-vascular System	Increases blood flow volume, especially coronary artery
hu ji sheng Cirsium japonicum	Cardio-vascular System	Dilates and increases blood flow volume of coronary vessels Significantly reduces heart rate Significantly lowers myocardial oxygen consumption Significantly lowers blood pressure
xu chang qing Cynanchum paniculatum	Cardio-vascular System	Lowers blood pressure
xue lian Saussurea laniceps	Smooth Muscle	Inhibits movements of isolated intestines
	Cardio-vascular System	Cardiac tonic
zu shi ma	Cardio-vascular System	Reduces blood pressure
fu she Agkistrodon acutus	Cardio-vascular System	Dilates blood vessels

5. Dampness Dissipating Aromatics

Herb Name	Pharmaceutical Functions	
	Organ Function	**Descriptions**
Cang zhu Atractylodes lancea	Digestive System	Increases bile secretions Anti-ulcerative, inhibits volume of gastric juice, gastric acidity and pepsin activity
hou po Magnolia officinalis	Digestive System	Inhibits gastric acid secretions caused by stress
	Smooth Muscle	At high dosages, excites isolated intestinal canal and bronchi, at low dosages, takes on inhibitory effect
huo xiang Agastache rugosa	Digestive System	Relaxes spasms of isolated ileum Inhibits spontaneous activities of duodenal smooth muscle Inhibits advancing function of gastrointestinal smooth muscle

6. Diuretics

Herb Name	Pharmaceutical Functions	
	Organ Function	**Descriptions**
ze xie Alisma plantago-aquatica	Cardio-vascular System	Lowers blood pressure Increases blood flow volume of coronary artery Lowers cardiac output and heart rate
yi yi ren Coix lacrymajobi	Cardio-vascular System	Inhibits isolated heart Reduces heart rate and lowers amplitude of contraction Temporarily lowers blood pressure
che qian cao Plantago asiatica	Respiratory System	Antagonises the excitatory effect on isolated tracheae caused by histamine or acetylchloride choline
bian xu Polygonum aviculare	Digestive System	Promotes bile secretions
	Cardio-vascular System	Temporarily lowers blood pressure

Herb Name	Pharmaceutical Functions	
	Organ Function	**Descriptions**
qu mai Dianthus superbus	Smooth Muscle	Significantly excites isolated intestines or intestinal canal in situ Increases intestinal peristalsis
	Cardio-vascular System	Inhibits isolated heart Lowers blood pressure
yu mi xu Zea mays	Cardio-vascular System	Lowers blood pressure
jin qian cao Ocimum basilicum	Digestive System	Promotes bile secretions
guang jin qian cao Ocimum basilicum (Guanzhou)	Digestive System	Increases bile flow volume
	Cardio-vascular System	Increases blood flow volume in coronary vessels Reduces heart rate, lowers blood pressure
hai jin sha Lygodium japonicum	Digestive System	Promotes bile secretions
yin chen Artemisia capillaris	Digestive System	Promotes bile secretions
ze xi Alisma plantago-aquatica	Smooth Muscle	Excites isolated small intestines Dilates isolated tracheae
di er cao Hypericum japonicum	Smooth Muscle	Increases rhythmic contraction of isolated intestines
	Cardio-vascular System	Slightly lower blood pressure

7. Interior Warming

Herb Name	Pharmaceutical Functions	
	Organ Function	**Descriptions**
fu zi Aconitum carmichaeli	Cardio-vascular System	Cardiac tonic Increases blood flow volume of coronary vessels Dilates blood vessels Reduces blood pressure
	Smooth Muscle	Excites isolated intestinal canal
rou gui Cinnamo-mum cassia	Digestive System	Anti-ulcerative Significantly inhibits intestinal peristalsis
wu zhu yu Evodia rutaecarpa	Digestive System	Excites isolated intestines at low dosages while significantly inhibits contraction at high dosages Anti-ulcerative
	Cardio-vascular System	Lowers blood pressure
gan jiang Zingiber officinalis	Digestive System	Tends to inhibit stress ulcer Significantly inhibits secretions of gastric juice Inhibits isolated intestinal movements Slows down peristalsis Increases bile secretions
	Cardio-vascular System	Increases blood pressure initially followed by reducing blood pressure
hua jiao Zanthoxylum bungeanum	Digestive System	Significantly inhibits ulcer; At low dosages excites isolated small intestines while at large dosages, inhibits large intestines

Herb Name	Pharmaceutical Functions	
	Organ Function	**Descriptions**
bi bo Piper longum	Cardio-vascular System	Lowers blood pressure, relaxes coronary vessels
	Smooth Muscle	Significantly relaxes intestinal smooth muscle
	Digestive System	Anti-ulcerative Significantly inhibits volume of gastric juice, total acidity of gastric juice
bi cheng qie Piper cubeba	Digestive System	Anti-ulcerative Promotes bile secretions Inhibits gastrointestinal peristalsis
	Cardio-vascular System	Lowers blood pressure
ding xiang Syzygium aromaticum	Digestive System	Promotes secretions of gastric juice Anti-ulcerative Inhibits movements of intestinal movements Promotes bile secretions
gao liang jiang Alpinia officinarum	Digestive System	Promotes secretions of gastric juice Increase total acid output in gastric juice Excites movements of isolated intestinal canal
xiao hui xiang Foeniculu vulgare	Digestive System	Excites contraction of isolated intestines Anti-ulcerative Promotes bile secretions
	Smooth Muscle	Relaxes smooth muscle in tracheae

8. Qi Activating

Herb Name	Pharmaceutical Functions	
	Organ Function	Descriptions
zhi shi Citri aurantii	Cardio-vascular System	Increases blood pressure Slightly increase blood flow volume in coronary vessels Significantly increases myocardial contractive Reduces heart rate Increases cardiac output
	Smooth Muscle	Extracts increases spontaneous movements of isolated intestinal canals Injection inhibits contraction of isolated intestinal smooth muscle and peristalsis of intestines in situ
zhi ke Citri aurantii	Smooth Muscle	Water decoction inhibits intestinal canal Gastrogavage of 100% water decoction promotes gastrointestinal peristalsis
chen pi Citri reticulatae	Smooth Muscle	Significantly inhibits smooth muscle contraction of isolated ileum
	Cardio-vascular System	Increases blood pressure
qing pi Citri reticula-tae viridae	Smooth Muscle	Inhibits smooth muscle contraction of isolated intestinal canal Antagonises bronchial and tracheal contraction induced by histamine Relaxes isolated tracheae and
	Cardio-vascular System	Increases blood pressure
xiang fu Cyperi rotundi	Cardio-vascular System	Lowers blood pressure Cardiac tonic, reduces heart rate
	Smooth Muscle	Inhibits isolated intestines Protects bronchial spasms caused by histamine

Herb Name	Pharmaceutical Functions	
	Organ Function	**Descriptions**
tu mu xiang Elecampane inulae	Smooth Muscle	Inhibits isolated intestines Lowers overactive movements and secretions of small intestine
chen xiang Aquilariae resinatum	Smooth Muscle	Inhibits spontaneous contraction of isolated ielum Relives spasms of intestinal smooth muscle
	Cardio-vascular System	Lowers blood pressure
wu yao Linderae strychnifoliae	Digestive System	Has bi-directional actions on gastrointestinal smooth muscle Increases secretions of digestive juice
chuan lian zi Meliae toosendan	Smooth Muscle	Excites tension and contraction of in situ or isolated intestinal smooth muscle
mu xiang Aucklandiae lappae	Digestive System	Different ingredients have different functions, some have anti-ulcerative function and promotes intestinal movements while others inhibits intestinal movements
	Cardio-vascular System	Inhibits the heart Different ingredients can increase or lower blood pressure
mei gui hua Rosae rugosae	Digestive System	Promotes bile secretions
fo shou Citri sarcodactylis	Smooth Muscle	Inhibits intestinal spasms Antagonises tracheal contraction caused by histamine
	Cardio-vascular System	Significantly increases blood flow volume in coronary vessels Inhibits the heart Lowers blood pressure

Herb Name	Pharmaceutical Functions	
	Organ Function	**Descriptions**
gan song Nardostach-yos	Cardio-vascular System	Lowers blood pressure
	Smooth Muscle	Relieves spasms of intestinal and tracheal smooth muscle

9. Digestive

Herb Name	Pharmaceutical Functions	
	Organ Function	**Descriptions**
lai fu zi Raphani sativi	Cardio-vascular System	Lowers blood pressure
	Smooth Muscle	Increases amplitude of contraction in isolated intestines
ji nei jin Endothelium corneum gigeriae galli	Digestive System	Increases secretions and acidity of gastric juice
ji shi teng Paederiae scandens	Cardio-vascular System	Lowers blood pressure
	Smooth Muscle	Inhibits contraction of isolated intestinal muscle
shan zha Crataegi	Cardio-vascular System	Increases blood flow volume of coronary vessels Cardiac tonic Lowers blood pressure

10. Anthelminthic and Antimalarial

Herb Name	Pharmaceutical Functions	
	Organ Function	**Descriptions**
ku lian pi Meliae radicis	Smooth Muscle	Excites intestinal smooth muscle
bing lang Arecae catechu	Digestive System	Excites isolated or in situ gallbladder, Induces strong contraction of gallbladder
wu mei Pruni mume	Smooth Muscle	Inhibits isolated intestines Relaxes Oddi's sphincter Promotes gallbladder contraction and bile discharging

11. Haemostatics

Herb Name	Pharmaceutical Functions	
	Organ Function	**Descriptions**
da ji Cirsii japonici	Cardio-vascular System	Lowers blood pressure
xiao ji Cephalano-ploris	Cardio-vascular System	Increases blood pressure Excites isolated heart
	Smooth Muscle	Inhibits intestinal smooth muscle Contracts bronchial smooth muscle
di yu Sanguisorbae officinalis	Cardio-vascular System	At low dosages increases contraction of isolated heart, reduces heart rate and increases cardiac output; takes on inhibitory effects at large dosage
	Smooth Muscle	At low dosages, decreases contraction of isolated intestinal smooth muscle; at high dosages, increases intestinal contraction

Herb Name	Pharmaceutical Functions	
	Organ Function	**Descriptions**
huai hua Sophorae Japonicae immaturus	Smooth Muscle	Lowers tension of smooth muscles in intestinal tract and bronchi
	Cardio-vascular System	Different ingredients has different functions, some slightly excite the heart, increase myocardial contractive and heart rate, some reduces heart rate Temporarily lowers blood pressure
xian he cao Agrimoniae pilosae	Cardio-vascular System	Increases blood pressure Contracts blood vessels in the organs
	Smooth Muscle	Different ingredients have different functions, inhibitory or excitatory
san qi Pseudogin-seng	Cardio-vascular System	Increases blood flow volume of coronary vessels Reduces heart rate, lowers blood pressure Lowers myocardial oxygen consumption
fu long gan Terra flava usta	Digestive System	Stops vomiting by inhibiting and anaesthetising gastrointestinal nerve ends
ai ye Artemisiae argyi	Respiratory System	Anti-asthmatic by relieving tracheal smooth muscle
	Digestive System	Promotes bile flow volume
	Cardio-vascular System	Inhibits the heart
dan shen Salviae miltiorrhizae	Cardio-vascular System	Increases blood flow volume in coronary vessel Inhibits cardiac contraction, decreases energy consumption
chuan xiong Ligustici wallichii	Cardio-vascular System	Increases blood flow volume in coronary vessel Inhibits blood vessel contraction
	Smooth Muscle	Inhibits contraction of small intestine

12. Blood-Circulation Activating and Blood-Stasis Removing

<table>
<tr><th rowspan="2">Herb Name</th><th colspan="2">Pharmaceutical Functions</th></tr>
<tr><th>Organ Function</th><th>Descriptions</th></tr>
<tr><td>yan hu suo
Corydalis</td><td>Cardio-vascular System</td><td>Increases blood flow volume in isolated coronary vessels
Lowers blood pressure</td></tr>
<tr><td>yi mu cao
Leonuri heterophylli</td><td>Cardio-vascular System</td><td>Dilates coronary artery, significantly increases blood flow volume in coronary vessels
Reduces heart rate</td></tr>
<tr><td>hong hua
Carthami tinctorii</td><td>Cardio-vascular System</td><td>Slightly excites the heart
Increases blood flow volume of coronary vessels
Reduces heart rate</td></tr>
<tr><td>jiang huang
Curcumae longae</td><td>Digestive System</td><td>Increases bile generation and secretion</td></tr>
<tr><td rowspan="2">hu zhang
Polygoni cuspidati</td><td>Cardio-vascular System</td><td>Lowers blood pressure</td></tr>
<tr><td>Respiratory System</td><td>Antiasthmatic
Antagonises tracheal contraction induced by histamine</td></tr>
<tr><td rowspan="2">yin xing ye
Ginkgo bilobae</td><td>Cardio-vascular System</td><td>Increases blood flow volume of coronary vessels</td></tr>
<tr><td>Smooth Muscle</td><td>Relieves spasms of isolated intestinal canal
Relaxes bronchial smooth muscle</td></tr>
<tr><td>ru xiang
Gummi olibanum</td><td>Smooth Muscle</td><td>Significantly inhibits movements of isolated intestines</td></tr>
</table>

13. Expectorants, Antitussive and Antiasthmatic

Herb Name	Pharmaceutical Functions: Organ Function	Pharmaceutical Functions: Descriptions
ban xia Pinelliae ternatae	Digestive System	Stops vomiting
	Cardio-vascular System	Temporarily lowers blood pressure
xuan fu hua Inulae britannica	Respiratory System	Antiasthmatic Antagonises isolated bronchial spasm induced by histamine
chuan bei mu Bulbus fritiliariae cirrhosae	Cardio-vascular System	Lowers blood pressure
	Smooth Muscle	Inhibits isolated intestines
zhe bei mu Bulbus fritillariae thunbergii	Cardio-vascular System	Reduces heart rate Lowers blood pressure
gua lou Trichosanthis krilowii	Digestive System	Anti-ulcerative Significantly lowers secretions and concentrations of gastric acid
tian zhu huang Concretio silicea bambusae T.	Cardio-vascular System	Reduces heart rate Slightly lowers blood pressure
kun bu Laminariae seu eckloniae	Cardio-vascular System	Lowers blood pressure
huang yao zi Dioscoreae bulbiferae	Smooth Muscle	Inhibits isolated intestines

Herb Name	Pharmaceutical Functions	
	Organ Function	Descriptions
pang da hai Scaphii lychnophori	Cardio-vascular System	Lowers blood pressure
ma dou ling Aristolochiae contorta	Respiratory System	Antiasthmatic, antagonises bronchial spasm induced by histamine
kuan dong hua Tussilaginis farfarae	Respiratory System	Slightly Antiasthmatic
	Smooth Muscle	Inhibits gastrointestinal smooth muscle
bai bu Stemonae	Respiratory System	Antiasthmatic, antagonises tracheal spasm induced by histamine
pi pa ye Eriobotryae japonicae	Respiratory System	Antiasthmatic
sang bai pi Mori albae radicis	Cardio-vascular System	Lowers blood pressure Inhibits isolated heart
	Smooth Muscle	Significantly increases gastrointestinal movements
yang jin hua Daturae metelis	Respiratory System	Increases respiration rate Antagonises smooth muscle contraction induced by acetylcholine or histamine
	Cardio-vascular System	Lowers blood pressure
	Digestive System	Inhibits ulcers Significantly inhibits volume of gastric juice, gastric acidity and output of total acid, lowers pepsin activity
ting li zi Descurainiae seu lepidii	Cardio-vascular System	Cardiac tonic

14. Tranquilizers

Herb Name	Pharmaceutical Functions: Organ Function	Pharmaceutical Functions: Descriptions
suan zao ren Zizyphi spinosae	Cardio-vascular System	Lowers blood pressure Cardiac tonic
yuan zhi Polygalae tenuifoliae	Cardio-vascular System	Lowers blood pressure
ling zhi Ganoderma-tus	Cardio-vascular System	Cardiac tonic
	Smooth Muscle	Inhibits smooth muscle activities of isolated ileum
ye jiao teng Polygoni multiflori	Smooth Muscle	Increases tension and contraction amplitude of small intestine muscle
	Cardio-vascular System	Lowers blood pressure

15. Liver Calming

Herb Name	Pharmaceutical Functions: Organ Function	Pharmaceutical Functions: Descriptions
di long Lumbricus	Respiratory System	Antiasthmatic, dilates bronchi
	Cardio-vascular System	Lowers blood pressure
gou teng Ramulus cum uncis uncariae	Cardio-vascular System	Lowers blood pressure Inhibits the heart
	Respiratory System	Antiasthmatic

Herb Name	Pharmaceutical Functions	
	Organ Function	Descriptions
tian ma Gastrodiae elatae	tian ma Gastrodiae Elatae	Slightly reduces heart rate Increases cardiac output Lowers blood pressure
bai ji li Tribulli terrestris	Cardio-vascular System	Lowers blood pressure Dilates coronary vessels Reduces heart rate
jue ming zi Cassiae	Cardio-vascular System	Lowers blood pressure
quan xie Buthus martensi	Cardio-vascular System	Reduces heart rate
wu gong Scolopendra subspinipes	Cardio-vascular System	Lowers blood pressure
luo bu ma Apocyni veneti	Cardio-vascular System	Reduces heart rate Lowers blood pressure

16. Analeptics

Herb Name	Pharmaceutical Functions	
	Organ Function	Descriptions
su he xiang Styrax liquidis	Cardio-vascular System	Reduces heart rate
shi chang pu Acori graminei	Digestive System	Promotes secretions of digestive juice Relieves smooth muscle spasms of intestinal canal
	Cardio-vascular System	Increases blood flow volume of coronary vessel
	Respiratory System	Antiasthmatic, dilates bronchi

17. Tonics

Herb Name	Pharmaceutical Functions	
	Organ Function	Descriptions
ren shen Panax ginseng	Cardio-vascular System	Cardiac tonic
dang shen Codonopsis pilosula	Cardio-vascular System	Lowers blood pressure
	Digestive System	Increases tension of isolated small intestines Partly antagonises increased gastric movements induced by stress Significantly inhibits basic gastric secretions
huang qi Astragalus membrana-ceus	Cardio-vascular System	Lowers blood pressure
bai zhu Atractylodes macrocephala	Digestive System	Bi-directionally affects intestinal canal Significantly decreases gastric juice volume, increase its ph and lowers pepsin activity
gan cao Glycyrrhiza uralensis	Digestive System	Anti-ulcerative Relieves spasms of gastric smooth muscle
shan yao Dioscorea opposita	Smooth Muscle	Restores normal rhythm of intestinal canals
ci wu jia Eleutherococ-cus senticosus	Cardio-vascular System	Lowers blood pressure temporarily
lu rong Cervus nippon	Cardio-vascular System	Transitorily lowers blood pressure
	Digestive System	Anti-ulcerative, inhibits secretions of gastric acid
yin yang huo Epimedium sagittatum	Cardio-vascular System	Increases myocardial contractive Increases blood flow volume of coronary vessels Lowers blood pressure

Herb Name	Pharmaceutical Functions	
	Organ Function	**Descriptions**
bu gu zhi Psoralea corylifolia	Cardio-vascular System	Increases blood flow volume of coronary vessels
tu si zi Cuscuta chinensis	Cardio-vascular System	Increases myocardial contractive Lowers blood pressure
dong chong xia cao Cordyceps sinensis	Cardio-vascular System	Lowers blood pressure
	Respiratory System	Antiasthmatic
du zhong Eucommia ulmoides	Cardio-vascular System	Lowers blood pressure
yi zhi ren Alpinia oxyphylla	Smooth Muscle	Inhibits iliac contraction
	Cardio-vascular System	Cardiac tonic
ge jie Gekko gecko	Respiratory System	Antiasthmatic, directly relaxes tracheal smooth muscle
sha yuan zi Astragalus complanatus	Cardio-vascular System	Lowers blood pressure Reduces heart rate
suo yang Cynomorium songaricum	Digestive System	Causes abnormal intestinal functions with the increase of dosage
she chuang zi Cnidium monnier	Respiratory System	Antiasthmatic, dilates bronchi
dang gui Angelica sinensis	Cardio-vascular System	Dilates coronary vessel Increases blood flow volume of coronary vessel Lowers blood pressure

Herb Name	Pharmaceutical Functions	
	Organ Function	**Descriptions**
dang gui Angelica sinensis	Respiratory System	Antiasthmatic, relaxes bronchial smooth muscle
he shou wu Polygonum multiflorum	Cardio-vascular System	Reduces heart rate
mai dong Ophiopogon japonicus	Cardio-vascular System	Increases myocardial contractive Reduces heart rate
bei sha shen Glehnia littoralis	Cardio-vascular System	At low dosages increases myocardial contractive of isolated heart, takes on inhibitor effect with the increase of dosage
gou qi zi Lycium barbarum	Cardio-vascular System	Lowers blood pressure Inhibits heart
	Smooth Muscle	Excites intestinal canal
nu zhen zi Ligustrum lucidum	Cardio-vascular System	Increases blood flow volume of coronary vessel Inhibits myocardial contractive
huang jing Polygonatum sibiricum	Cardio-vascular System	Lowers blood pressure Increases myocardial contractive
yu zhu Polygonatum odoratum	Cardio-vascular System	Cardiac tonic Slightly lowers blood pressure or slowly increase blood pressure in different animals
bai he Lilium brownii	Respiratory System	Antiasthmatic, antagonises asthma caused by histamine
nan sha shen Adenophora stricta	Cardio-vascular System	Cardiac tonic
mo han lian Eclipta prostrata	Cardio-vascular System	Increases blood flow volume of coronary vessel

18. Astringents

<table>
<tr><th rowspan="2">Herb Name</th><th colspan="2">Pharmaceutical Functions</th></tr>
<tr><th>Organ Function</th><th>Descriptions</th></tr>
<tr><td rowspan="2">wu wei zi
Schisandra chinensis</td><td>Cardio-vascular System</td><td>Increases blood flow volume of coronary vessel
Lowers blood pressure</td></tr>
<tr><td>Digestive System</td><td>Anti-ulcerative
Inhibits iliac contraction
Promotes bile secretions
Inhibits gastric contraction</td></tr>
<tr><td>rou dou kou
Myristica fragrans</td><td>Digestive System</td><td>Increases gastric juice secretions
Stimulates gastrointestinal peristalsis at low dosages, while takes on inhibitory effect at large dosages</td></tr>
</table>

Adaptogens

Adaptogens restore normality to an organism under environmental pressure (stress) and has a normalising influence on a pathological state, independent of the nature of the state. An adaptogen must be innocuous and not disturb body function at a normal level (Panossian, 2004). There is increasing evidence that prolonged exposure to stressful life events and depression are both related to significant behavioural, endocrinological and neurobiological changes in human and animal subjects and adaptogens are a critical therapeutic approach..

Adaptogens vs. Stimulants

	Stimulants	Adaptogens
Recovery after Physical Loading	Low	High
Energy Depletion	Yes	No
Performance Under Stress	Decrease	Increase
Survival Under Stress	Decrease	Increase
Quality of Arousal	Poor	Good
Insomnia	Yes	No
Side Effects	Yes	No
DNA/RNA and Protein Synthesis	Decrease	Increase

(Panossian 2003)

Adaptogens are botanicals, which are bi-directional in activity. They restore 'normalcy' but have no specific impact on a healthy, balanced organism.

Adaptogen Herbs:
ren shen (panax ginseng)
Cardiovascular System
Cardiac tonic
Adaptogenic
Increases resistance to stress and ageing and the adaptogenic properties of ginseng are believed to be due to its effects on hypothalamic - pituitary - adrenal axis, resulting in elevated plasma corticotrophin and corticosteroids levels (Nocerino et al, 2000).

dang shen (codonopsis pilosula)
Cardiovascular System
Lowers blood pressure
Digestive System
Increases tension of isolated small intestines
Partly antagonises increased gastric movements induced by stress
Significantly inhibits basic gastric secretions

huang qi (astragalus membranaceus)
Cardiovascular System
Lowers blood pressure
Protects against free radical damage and inhibits cardiac lipid peroxidation
Immunity
Stimulates immunity and enhances production of immunoglobulins
Promotes metabolism of serum liver proteins, growth of antibodies and increases white blood cells (Wilson-Hare, 1997).

bai zhu (atractylodes macrocephala)
Digestive System
Bi-directionally affects intestinal canal
Significantly decreases gastric juice volume, increase its ph and lowers pepsin activity

jiao gu lan (gynostemma pentaphyllum)
Endocrine System
Increases ACTH levels and is an antioxidant (Chen & Chen, p. 854).

It enhances the antioxidant enzyme activity in some tissues of exhausted mice, and to a certain extent inhibits the lipid peroxidation damage (Wang & Chi, 2008).
It increases liver glucose (LG) and muscle glucose (MG) content, while AKT/PKB (protein kinase B) enzyme and lactate dehydrogenase (LDH) activity decreased significantly (Long et al, 2008).

xi yang shen (panax quinquefolius)
Significantly prolongs the swimming time of yin-deficiency Jimpy mice, compared with model control group, the high-dose group and the low-dose group demonstrate a significant difference (Li et al, 2007).
Anti-oxidation acidity may related to the increase of the glutathione peroxidase (GSH-Px) and superoxidedismutase (SOD) activities. Decreases LH (luteinising hormone) levels (as does melatonin) and increases serum ceruloplasmin (CP) oxidase activity (a measure of oestrogenic activity in the liver) (Göçmen et al, 2008).
Prevented the rise of serum ALT activity, inhibited MDA formation and increased GSH—PX activities. Xi yang shen alleviated CCl_4—induced liver toxicity in rats (Zhao, 1997).

xi yang shen & jiao gu lan
(panax quinquefolius & gynostemma pentaphyllum)
Both xi yang shen and jiao gu lan have a CNS depressive effect, they increase energy and endurance, stimulates immunity, has an anti-ageing effect while reducing stress levels. Gynostemma has a particularly strong sedative effect (Chen & Chen, p. 842).

Rhodiola rosea
3% rosavin and 1% salidroside
The extract significantly, but not dose-dependently, induced antidepressant-like, adaptogenic, anxiolytic-like and stimulating effects in mice.
This study thus provides evidence of the efficacy of R. rosea extracts after a single administration, and indicates the adaptogenic

and stimulating effects of R. rosea extracts (Perfumi & Mattioli, 2008).

Standardised 3% rosavin and 1% salidroside extraction
Chronic administration of R. rosea results in potent inhibition of the behavioural and physiological changes induced by chronic exposure to stressors (Mattioli et al, 2009). It has antidepressant, adaptogenic, anxiolytic, nociceptive and locomotor activities at doses of 10, 15 and 20 mg/kg, using predictive behavioural tests and animal models (Perfumi & Mattioli, 2008).

hou po (magnolia officinalis)
Standardised Magnolol and Honokiol (M&H) extract.
Hou po disperses the middle jiao and dries Damp. It inhibits the CNS but stimulates respiration (Chen & Chen, p.366).
Honokiol selectively induces an anxiolytic effect with less liability of eliciting motor dysfunction and sedation or disinhibition (Kuribara, 1998). M & H interact with GABA-A receptors in rat brain in vitro. The potentiation of GABAergic neurotransmission by M & H is probably involved in their previously reported anxiolytic and central depressant effects (Squires et al, 1999).

REFERENCES

Beauchaine, T. P., Gatzke-Kopp, L. and Mead, H. K. (2007). Polyvagal Theory and Developmental Psychopathology: Emotion Dysregulation and Conduct Problems from Preschool to Adolescence. *Biol Psychol, 74*(2), 174–184.

Berthoud H-R, Neuhuber WL. (2000). Functional and chemical anatomy of the afferent vagal system. *Auton Neurosci* 85, 1–17.

Cohen, S. & Rodriguez, M.S. *Pathways linking affective disturbances and physical disorders.* Health Psychology. Vol 14(5), Sep 1995, 374-380. doi: 10.1037/0278-6133.14.5.374

Coulter, H. (1994a). Empiricism vs. Rationalism in Medicine. *The Journal of Orthomolecular Medicine, 9*(3).

Coulter, H. (1994b). *Divided Legacy: A History of the Schism in Medical Thought; Vol IV, Twentieth-Century Medicine, The Bacteriological Era.* North Atlantic Books: California.

Cozolino, L. *The Neuroscience of Human Relationships.* WW Norton & Co. 2006. NY

Esler, M., Turbott, J., Schwarz, R., Leonard, P., Bobik, A., Skews, H., Jackman, G. (1982). The peripheral kinetics of norepiniphrine in depressive illness. Arch Gen *Psychiatry, 39,* 285–300.

Gao, Ming 高明. (1996). *Commentaries on the Silk Scroll Book of Laozi, Boshu Laozi Xiaozhu* 帛書老子校註. Beijing: Zhonghua Shuju.

Gellhorn, E. (1967). *Principles of Autonomic-Somatic Integrations.* Minneapolis: University of Minnesota Press.

Ghia, J.E., Blennerhassett, P., Kumar-Ondiveeran, H., Verdu, E.F., and Collins, S.M. (2006). The vagus nerve: a tonic inhibitory influence associated with inflammatory bowel disease in a murine model, *Gastroenterology 131*(4), 1122–1130

Guo, Qingpan 郭慶藩. 1997. *An Elucidation on Zhuangzi, Zhuangzi Jishi* 莊子集釋. Beijing: Zhonghua Shuju.

Habib, K. E., Gold, P. W., Chrousos, G. P. (2001). Neuroendocrinology of Stress. *Endocrinology and metabolism clinics of North America*, 30, 695-728.

Hellhammer, D.H., and Klingmann, P.O. (2008). *Serotonergic and Parasympathetic Disorders.* Hellhammer DH, Hellhammer J (eds): *Stress. The Brain-Body Connection. Key Issues in Mental Health.* Basel, Karger, 174, 91–105.

Kaptchuk, T.J. (1987). The Culture, History and Discourse of Oriental Medicine. *Journal of Chinese Medicine, 24*, 7-17.

Kleinman, A. (1987). Anthropology and psychiatry. The role of culture in cross-cultural research on illness. *Br J Psychiatry,* 151, 447-54.

Kuribara, H., Stavinoha, W.B., Maruyama, Y. (1998). Honokiol, a putative anxiolytic agent extracted from magnolia bark. *Journal of Pharm Pharmacol,* 50(7), 819-26.

Lao, T.L. (1990). The Use Of The Sanjiao Theory In Clinical Acupuncture. *Journal Of Chinese Medicine* No, 34, 20-2.

Larre, C., and Vallee, E.R. (1992). *Heart Master Triple Heater.* London: Monkey Press.

Liu, Y.Q., Cheng, M.C., Wang, L.X., Zhao, N. & Xiao, H.B. (2008). Functional Analysis of Cultured Neural Cells for Evaluating Cold/Cool and Hot/Warm Natured Chinese Herbs. *The American Journal of Chinese Medicine,* 36(4) 771–781.

Long, B., Zhang, K., Hu, J., Zhou, Z., Zhou, X. (2008). Hai Nan Shi Fan Da Xue Xue Bao. *Zi Ran Ke Xue Ban,* 21(3), 334-37.

Ma, T., Tan, C., Zhang, H., Wang, M., Ding, W. & Li, S. (2010). Bridging the gap between traditional Chinese medicine and systems biology: the connection of Cold Syndrome and NEI network. *Mol. BioSyst*, 6, 613–619. DOI: 10.1039/b914024g.

Mateer, C.W. (1901–2). The meaning of the word shen. *Chinese Recorder* 3(2), 61–72, 107–16, 3(3), 71–79, 123–32.

Mattioli L, Funari C & Perfumi M. (2009). Effects of Rhodiola rosea L. extract on behavioural and physiological alterations induced by chronic mild stress in female rats. *Journal of Psychopharmacology*, 23(2), 130-142. (2009) DOI: 10.1177/0269881108089872

Mayer, E.A. (2000). The Neurobiology of Stress and Gastrointestinal Disease. *Gut*, 47, 861-869.

McCance K.L. (1998). Pathophysiology, *The Biological Basis for Disease in Adults and Children*, 3rd Ed. Mosby: St Louis.

MSSS. Accessed 04 / 10 http://publications.msss.gouv.qc.ca/acrobat/f/documentation/2009/09-235-12A_01.pdf <http://publications.msss.gouv.qc.ca/acrobat/f/documentation/2009/09-235-12A_01.pdf> .

Ng, G.A. Brack, K.E. and Coote, J.H. (2001). Effects of direct sympathetic and vagus nerve stimulation on the physiology of the whole heart--a novel model of isolated Langendorff perfused rabbit heart with intact dual autonomic innervation. *Experimental Physiology*, 86, 3, 319-329.

Nocerino, E., Amato, M. & Izzo, A.A. (2000). The aphrodisiac and adaptogenic properties of ginseng. *Fitoterapia*, 71(1), S1-S5. doi:10.1016/S0367-326X(00)00170-2.

Ou, B., Huang, D., Hampsch-Woodill, M., Flanagan, J.A. (2003).When east meets west: the relationship between yin-yang and anti-oxidation/oxidation. FASEB J, 17(2), 127-9.

Panossian, A.G. (2003). Adaptogens; Tonic Herbs for Fatigue and Stress. *Alternative and Complementary Therapies*. 9(6), 327-31. doi:10.1089/107628003322658610.

Perfumi, M. & Mattioli, L. Adaptogenic and central nervous system effects of single doses of 3% rosavin and 1% salidroside Rhodiola rosea L. extract in mice. *Phytotherapy Research*, 21(1), 37 - 43. DOI:10.1002/ptr.2013.

Pert, C. (1998). *Molecules of Emotion: the Science Behind Mindbody Medicine:* Simon and Schuster.

Porges, S.W. (1995). Orienting in a defensive world: Mammalian modifications of our evolutionary heritage. A Polyvagal Theory. *Psychophysiology*, 32, 301-318.

Porges, S. W. (1992). Vagal Tone: A Physiologic Marker of Stress Vulnerability. *Paediatrics*, 90, 498-504.

Porges, S.W. (1998). Love : An emergent property of the mammalian autonomic nervous system. *Psychoneuroendocrinology*, 23(8), 837-861.

Porges, S.W. (2001). Retrieved 01/09. http://stanleyrosenberg.com/english/articles/polyvagal_theory/

Porges, S. (1995). Cardiac vagal tone: A physiological index of stress. *Neuroscience & Biobehavioural Reviews*. 19(2), 225-33.

Rasul, F., Stansfeld, S.A., Hart, C.L., Gillis, C., Smith, G.D. (2003). Somatic symptoms and depression. Symposium abstracts / *Journal of Psychosomatic Research* 55, 111–129

Reale, G. (1990). A History of Ancient Philosophy: Plato and Aristotle. SUNY Press.

Robinson, L. (1990). Stress and anxiety. *Nursing Clinics of North America*, 25(4),

935-43.

Rogers, R.C., McTigue, D.M., and Hermann, G.E. (1996).Vagal control of digestion: Modulation by central neural and peripheral endocrine factors. *Neuroscience & Biobehavioral Reviews.* 20(1), 57-66.

Rose, J.D.R., Troughton, A.H., Harvey, J.S. and Smith, P.M. (1986). Depression and functional bowel disorders in gastrointestinal outpatients. *Gut,* 27, 1025-1028.

Schuessler, Axel. (2007). ABC Etymological Dictionary of Old Chinese. University of Hawaii Press.

Schwartz, B. I. (1985). *The World of Thought in Ancient China.* Cambridge, MA: Harvard University Press.

Simon, G.E., Von Korff, M., Saunders, K., Miglioretti, D.L., Crane, P.K., van Belle, G., Kessler, R.C. (2006). Association between obesity and psychiatric disorders in the US adult population. *Archives of General Psychiatry,* 63(7), 824-830.

Squires, R.F., Ai, J., Witt, M-R., Kahnberg, P., Saederup, E., Sterner, O. & Nielsen, M. (1999). Honokiol and Magnolol Increase the Number of [3H] Muscimol Binding Sites Three-Fold in Rat Forebrain Membranes In Vitro Using a Filtration Assay, by Allosterically Increasing the Affinities of Low-Affinity Sites. *Neurochemical Research,* 24(12), 1593-1602.

Standish, A., Enquist, L.W. and Schwaber, J.S. (1994). Innervation of the heart and its central medullary origin defined by viral tracing. *Science,* 263(5144), 232-4.

van der Greef, J., Stroobant, P. & van der Heijden, R. (2004). The role of analytical sciences in medical systems biology. *Current Opinion in Chemical Biology,* 8, 559–65. DOI 10.1016/j.cbpa.2004.08.013.

Wang, H-y., Chi, A-p. (2008) *Shi Ping Ke Xue,* 29(11), 616-18.

Wellwood, J. (1992). *Ordinary Magic.* Shambhala.

West TCM, Vancouver / Langley Canada. Retrieved 01/09. http://tcm.health-info.org/

Wilson-Hare, L.K. (1997). Surviving Stress. Dissertation.com <http://Dissertation.com> <http://Dissertation.com/> Boca Raton. http://scholar.google.com.au/scholar?cluster=10022948312930830006&hl=en&as_sdt=2000

Xu, X.Y., Li, L.H., Wu, L.S., Zhao, C.L., Lin, H.Y. (2002). *Zhongguo Zhong Yao Za Zhi,* 27(10), 771-3.

Yoshino, K. and Matsuoka, K. (2008). Correlation between mood during daily life and autonomic nervous system activity during sleep. Proceedings of Measuring Behaviour

INDEX

A

B

C

I

J

K

L

M

N

O

P

Q

R

S

T

Z

AUTHOR'S BIOGRAPHY

Daniel Weber is CEO of Panaxea Medical, an accomplished international lecturer and author. Daniel holds the Vice-Chairmanship in Oncology for the World Federation of Chinese Medicine Societies. Daniel has a BA in Acupuncture, a post-graduate diploma both in Somatic Psychotherapy and in Adult Education, a Master of Science degree in Chinese herbal medicine, and a PhD in Traditional Chinese Medicine. Daniel is also a registered psychotherapist (MPACFA).

Daniel is currently enrolled in a Doctor of Health Science at Charles Sturt University. Daniel has lectured in Australia, the UK and South Africa, Japan and China, and is a frequent lecturer in the United States. He is the author of 'Introduction to Integrative Oncology', 'Inflammation and the Seven Stochastic Events of Cancer', "Dui Yao' the Art of Formula Construction and the groundbreaking, first English language database on Chinese Herbs, published in 1992. His company, Panaxea is an innovative practitioner only complementary medicine manufacturer and distributor.